Drugs and Cosmetics Formulations

Drugs and Cosmetics Formulations

Ranjan Magazine
Plant Head—Manufacturing and Marketing
Sunny Allied Industries
Jammu
J&K

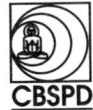

CBSPD

CBS Publishers & Distributors Pvt Ltd

New Delhi • Bengaluru • Chennai • Kochi • Kolkata • Lucknow • Mumbai
Hyderabad • Jharkhand • Nagpur • Patna • Pune • Uttarakhand

Drugs and Cosmetics Formulations

ISBN: 978-81-239-1994-2

First Edition : 2011
Reprint: 2014, 2019, 2023

Published by Satish Kumar Jain and produced by Varun Jain for
CBS Publishers & Distributors Pvt Ltd
4819/XI Prahlad Street, 24 Ansari Road, Daryaganj, New Delhi 110 002, India
Ph: 011-23289259, 23266861

Website: www.cbspd.com
e-mail: delhi@cbspd.com

Corporate Office: 204 FIE, Industrial Area, Patparganj, Delhi 110 092, India
Ph: 011-4934 4934   Fax: 011-4934 4935   e-mail: publishing@cbspd.com; publicity@cbspd.com

Branches

- **Bengaluru:** Seema House 2975, 17th Cross, KR Road, Banasankari 2nd Stage, Bengaluru 560 070, Karnataka, India
  Ph: +91-80-26771678/79   Fax: +91-80-26771680   e-mail: bangalore@cbspd.com
- **Chennai:** 7, Subbaraya Street, Shenoy Nagar, Chennai 600 030, Tamil Nadu, India
  Ph: +91-44-26680620, 26681266   Fax: +91-44-42032115   e-mail: chennai@cbspd.com
- **Kochi:** 42/1325, 1326, Power House Road, Opp KSEB, Power House, Ernakulam, Kochi 682 018, India
  Ph: +91-484-4059061–65   Fax: +91-484-4059065   e-mail: kochi@cbspd.com
- **Kolkata:** 147, Hind Ceramics Compound, 1st Floor, Nilgunj Road, Belghoria, Kolkata 700 056, West Bengal, India
  Ph: +91-33-25633055–56   e-mail: kolkata@cbspd.com
- **Lucknow:** Basement, Khushnuma Complex, 7-Meerabai Marg (behind Jawahar Bhawan), Lucknow 226 001, India
  Ph: +91-522-4000032   e-mail: tiwari.lucknow@cbspd.com
- **Mumbai:** PWD Shed, Gala no. 25/26, Ramchandra Bhatt Marg, Next to JJ Hospital Gate no. 2, Opp. Union Bank of India, Noorbaug Mumbai 400 009, Maharashtra, India
  Ph: +91-22-66661880/89   e-mail: mumbai@cbspd.com

Representatives

- **Hyderabad** 0-9885175004
- **Jharkhand** 0-9811541605
- **Nagpur** 0-9421945513
- **Patna** 0-9334159340
- **Pune** 0-9923910676
- **Uttarakhand** 0-9716462459

Printed at: Mudrak, Noida, UP

Preface

This is an important book in drugs and cosmetics formulations for the purpose of students, laboratory practice, pharmacists, formulators and the personnel in manufacturing sector. The chapters covers all aspects of drugs and cosmetics formulations like men, methods, machines, calculations, yields, formulations of allopathic medicines, ayurvedic medicines, herbal products, natural products, homeopathic medicines, images, appendices, teaching, R&D, production, marketing and product literature, which are most useful in daily needs.

For solid dosage forms excipients are needed in formulation due to machines and liquids need excipients because of flavour, smell, taste, stability, antioxidation process and preservative formulations. If kept unformulated, liquids will decompose, so one should stop losses. Semisolids need excipients due to antioxidation, preservatives, smell processes. Chemical and microbiological testing is needed for solid, liquid and semisolid products. Most of the drugs and cosmetics formulations are based on IP/BP/USP/WHO/ISO series/FDA test approvals.

Methods are written to calculate MRP calculation of pharmacy products.

Materials with pictures used in packing have been explained.

Lists of drug and cosmetics ingredients are written and explained.

Suggestions from all the readers are most welcome.

Ranjan Magazine
ranjan.magazine@gmail.com

Acknowledgements

I express my true thanks to my parents for writing this book on drugs and cosmetics formulations.

I also express true thanks to CBS Publishers & Distributors for their time and effort in publishing this edition.

Ranjan Magazine

Contents

Appendices

1 Uncoated, Dispersible and Coated Tablets Technologies

Fundamental principles of uncoated, dispersible tablets **/Coated tablet formulation

1. Weight of drug (in metric system) .... (Direct compression method)

2. Drug dry slugging (small pieces)

3. Dry granules .... (dry granulation method) .... Compression

4. Weight of excipients .... wet granulation method

5. Shifting (to shift raw material in polythene bags)

6. Milling (to make smaller particle)

7. Dispersible tablets** Sweetening agent milled sugar 97% w/w or aspartame 1% to 2%, colour ponceau 4 R 0.03% w/w and opicifier titanium dioxide 0.001% w/w, Flavour raspberry 0.21% w/w, Buffering agent citric acid 0.1% w/w.

8. (Wet granulation) .... wet mixing (starch paste~ + drug)~ binding agent starch paste = 120% w/v starch powder in cool water or 3 to 5% w/v, starch in RO water, then boiling at 60 degrees/CMC 2 to 4% w/v in cool RO water or acacia 1 to 2% w/v in boiling water at 60°C.

   **Binding agent ethanol 50% v/v and RO water 50% v/v to make polyvinylpyrrolidone K-30 paste 1 to 2% w/v

9. Wet material drying (at 60°C)

10. *Multi Mill:* Breaking big lumps

11. Drying at 60°C

12. Wet granulation (making wet granules)

13. Dry granulation (making dry granules at 60°C)

14. *Lubrication:* Dry mixing (mixing dry granules and anti-adhesive magnesium stearate 0.2 to 2% w/w, **Disintegrator starch powder 5 % to 10% w/w, lubricant talcum powder 0.2% to 5% w/w, diluent colloidal silicon dioxide 1% to 2%, surfactant sodium lauryl sulphate 0.01% to 0.05% w/w, other pharmaceutical excipients if needed)

15. Compression (to make uncoated tablets)

16. Coating (Film*, enteric ***, sugar) film coating* suspension, spray and drying at 35°C of film coating material hydroxypropyl methylcellulose 1% w/v in vehicle isopropyl alcohol 70% v/v, glidant talc 1% w/w, plasticizer triethyl citrate 0.5% w/w, opicifier titanium dioxide 0.001% w/v, colour ponceau 4 R 0.03% w/v, sustain release coating suspension, spray and drying at 35°C, hydroxypropyl methylcellulose 1% w/v, ethyl cellulose 0.5% w/v in vehicle isopropyl alcohol 70% v/v, glidant talc 1%, plasticizer triethyl citrate 0.5% w/w, opicifier titanium dioxide 0.001% w/v, colour ponceau 4 R 0.03% w/v, enteric coating ***suspension, spray and drying at 35°C of enteric coating cellulose acetate phthalate (soluble at pH > 6) 1% w/v in isopropyl alcohol 70% v/v, glidant talc 1% w/w, plasticizer triethyl citrate 0.5% w/w, colours ponceau 4 R 0.03% w/v and opicifier titanium dioxide 0.001% w/v sustain release coating can be controlled release coating or sodium CMC high viscosity 2 to 4 % w/v. Sugar coating contain solution of sugar syrup 68% w/v, citric acid 0.1% w/v, sodium benzoate 0.1% w/v, colour ponceau 4 R 0.1% w/v is sprayed on uncoated tablets and sugar coating tablets are dried at 60°C. All types of coating must be only 1 mm in thickness to avoid wastage and production loss during strip, blister and alu packing.

17. Packing (strip, blister, alu, 15 kg HMHDPE drums)
    Quality control and quality assurance for 20 tablets is:
    • Weight variation = Weight of tablet ± 5% in mg
    • Thickness = Size of tablet ± 5 % in mm
    • Hardness = 4 kg/cm². No tablet breaking while transport.

- Friability = Chamber rotation for 4 minutes @ 25 rpm. Weight loss limit not more than (NMT) 0.8 % w/w .

Clean tablets: No mobilile oil.

Rate of disintegration time: At 35°C uncoated tablets (within 30 minutes) must disintegrate and coated tablets (within 1 hour) must disintegrate and pass through the sieve.

Dissolution test time: 100% tablet must dissolve and weight of drug must be equivalent to the label claim by chemical analysis (within 1 hour)

Storage: Airtight packing.
Yield% = Obtained weight/supplied weight * 100.
Yield% must be above 92% to obtain profit in business.

Tablets produced by direct compression: Aspirin, chlorine, ferrous sulphate.

Tablets produce by dry granulation: Calcium lactate, riboflavin, alprazolam.

Tablets produced by wet granulation: Paracetamol, sodium bicarbonate. 70% of drugs are produced by wet granulation method.

Machines used

1. Sifter
2. Mass mixer
3. Hot air drier
4. Multi mill
5. Hammer mill or motar and pestle of iron
6. Oscillating granulator
7. Drum mixer
8. Tablet making machine
9. Coating pan
10. Tablet disintegration
11. Tablet dissolution machine
12. Tablet hardness tester
13. Tablet friability machine
14. Strip or blister machine

15. Batch printing machine
16. Label gumming machine
17. Taping and sealing cartons
18. Digital balance
19. Measuring cylinder
20. Compactor

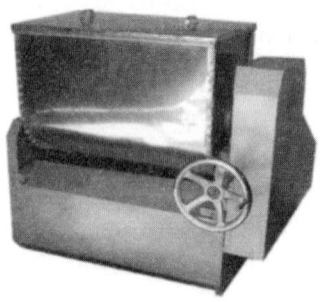

Mass mixer

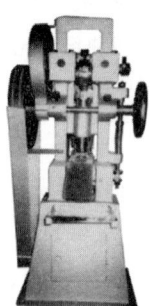

Tablet machine with
13 stations (die sets)

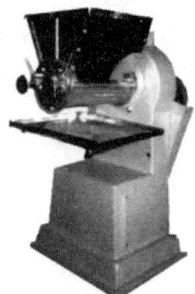

Oscillating
granulator

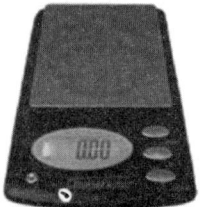

Digital balance for
weighing in milligrams

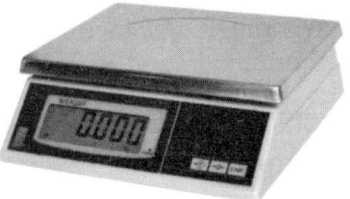

Digital balance for
weighing in kilograms

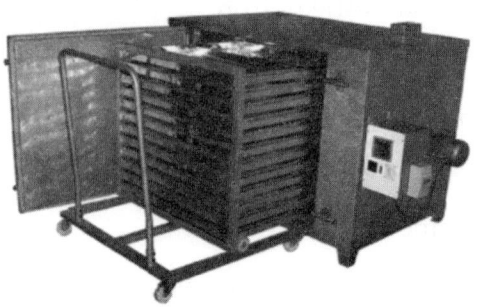

Drier 24 trays

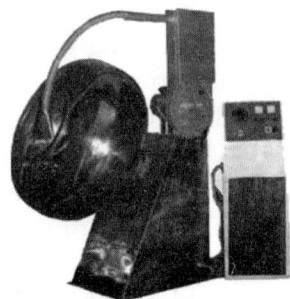

Coating pan for coating tablets

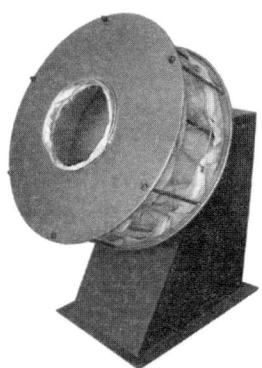

Polishing pan for sugar
coating tablets

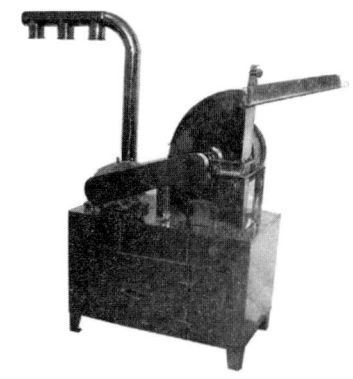

Hammer mill for milling hard materials like
herbal powder, homeopathic tablets

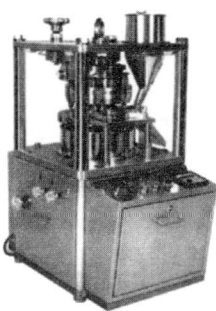

Rotary tablet machine with
51 stations

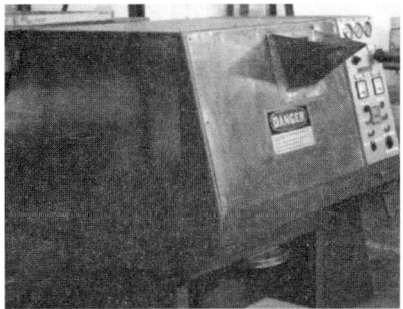

Roll compactor for dry granulation with
quality s.s 306

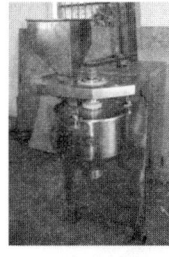

Multi mill for
wet granulation
of tablets

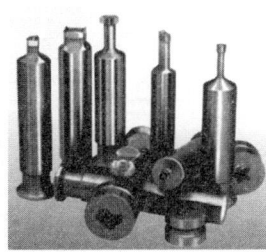

Punches and dies of
tablet machine

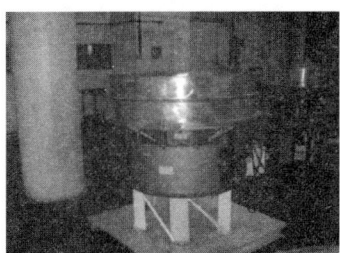

Sifter

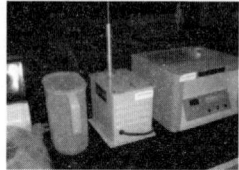
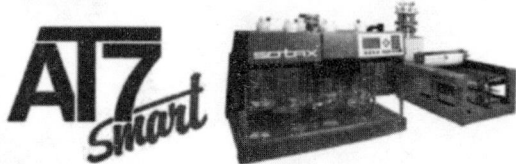

Disintegrator   Dissolution

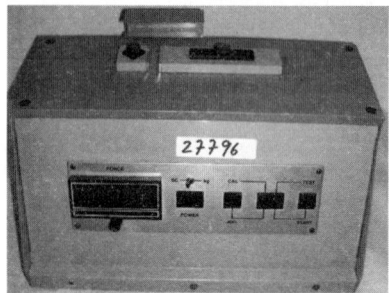
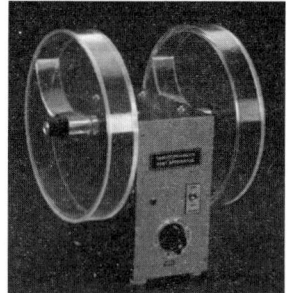

Tablet hardness tester   Friability

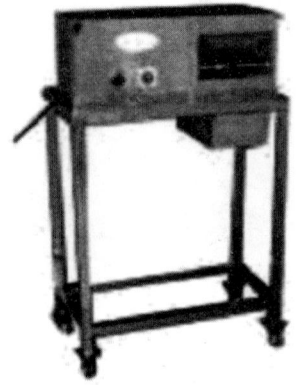
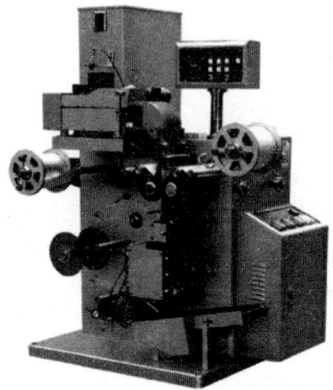

Tablet defoiler   Blister machine

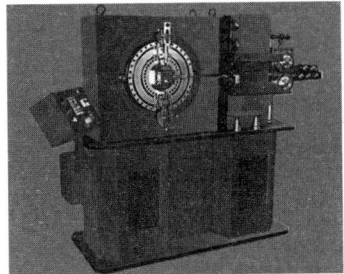

Strip machine

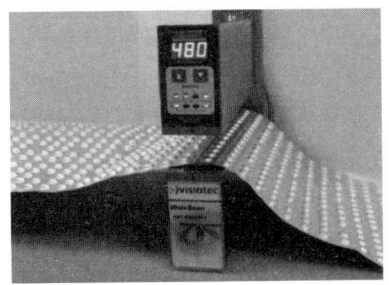

Pin hole detector

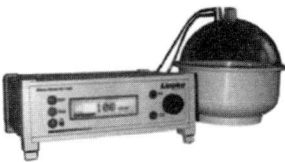

Blister leak tester

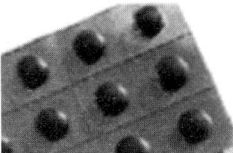

Blister pack of film coated tablets

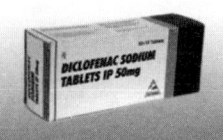

Show box

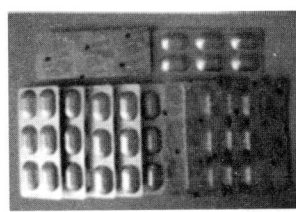

Alu pack of tablets

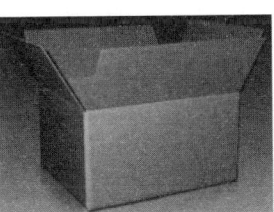

5 ply carton

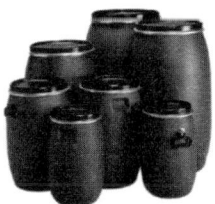

HMHDPE drums

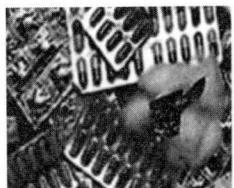

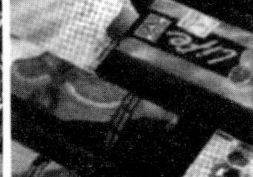

Strip and bister pack and show box

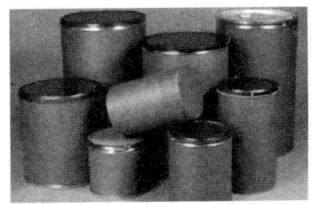

Fiber drums

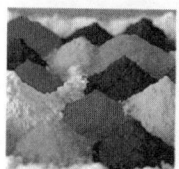 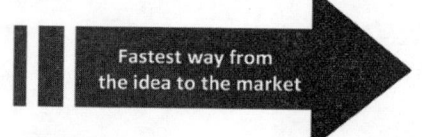

Dry powder to finished products

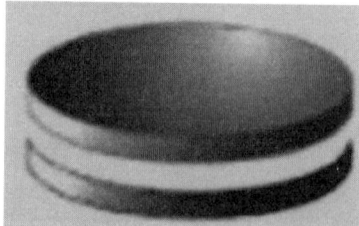

Bilayer tablet

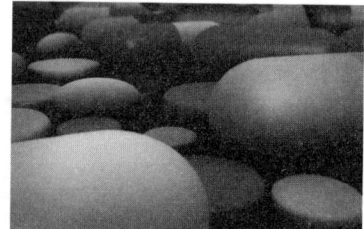

Uncoated, coated tablets and capsule

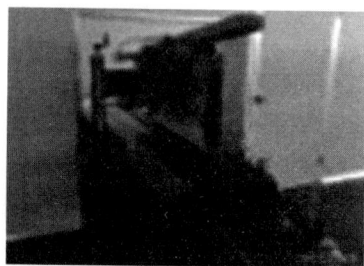

Carton sealing machine

2 Eye and Ear Drops Technology

Fundamental principles of eye/ear drops formulation

1. Weight of drug
2. Distilled water (vehicle) q.s.
3. Citric acid (buffering agent acidic) 0.5% w/v
4. Sodium chloride 0.9% w/w (tonicity)
5. Sodium EDTA 0.05% w/w (stablizer)
6. Methylparaben 0.08% w/w, propylparaben 0.04% w/w (preservative)

Mix and stir 1, 2, 3, 4, 5 and 6 in small volume. Now stir for 1 hour in the required volume and dissolve.

After sterility test, chemical test, progen test, leak test and clarity test, eye/ear drops are ready for packing in vials. Yield% must be greater than 99%.

Machines used

1. Stainless steel tank
2. Stirrer
3. Filter press
4. Volumetric liquid filling machine
5. Laminar flow machine
6. Batch printing machine
7. Label gumming machine
8. Taping and sealing machine
9. 20 litres tank containing formaldehyde and potassium permanganate
10. Digital balance
11. Measuring cylinder.

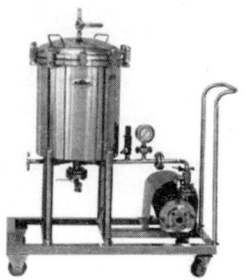

Filter press

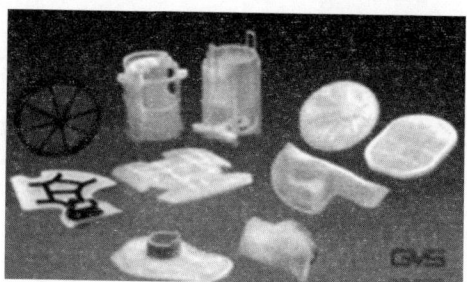

Nylon filters

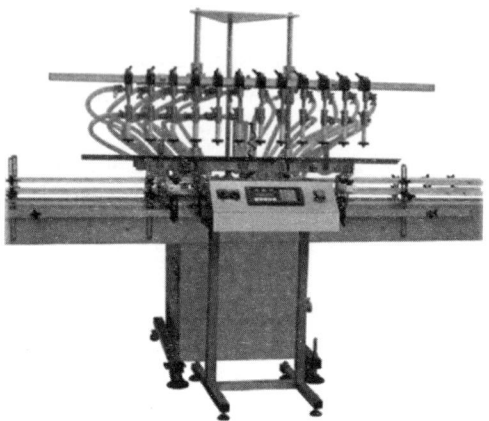

Automatic volumetric liquid filling machine

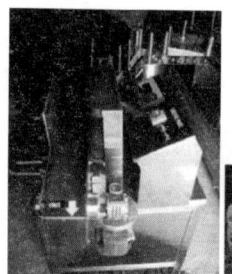

Label gumming machine

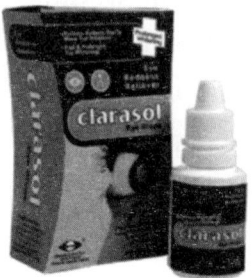

Bottle of eye/ ear drops

3 Analgesic Cream Formulations

Fundamental principles of analgesic cream formulation

1. Water phase
   a. Vehicle RO water = 8 litres
   b. Weight of analgesic drug like diclofenac, etc.
   c. Preservatives methyl paraben = 0.08% w/w (8 grams), propylparaben = 0.04% w/w (4 grams)
   d. Essence lavender oil (0.5%) = 50 ml
2. Oil phase
   a. Emollient mineral oil = 1 litre
   b. Emollient emulsifying wax stearic acid = 1 kg

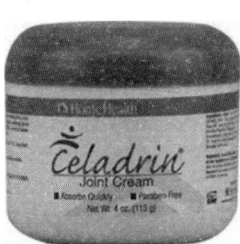

Analgesic cream

Method

Dissolve in water phase a, b, c. Boil/melt at 60°C water phase and oil phase separately. Now slowly mix oil phase in water phase at 60°C in emulsifier for 15 minutes. Mix lavender oil and emulsify for 5 minutes.

Analgesic cream is ready for packing in tubes. Yield% must be greater than 97%.

Machines used

1. Stainless steel tank
2. Emulsifier
3. Heater
4. Cream filling machine
5. Batch printing machine
6. Label gumming machine
7. Taping and sealing machine
8. Digital balance
9. Measuring cylinder

4   *Emulsion Formulation Technology*

Fundamental principles of emulsion formulation

Part A

Oil phase:
1. Emulsifying wax stearic acid = 500 gm
2. Mineral oil = 500 ml

Part B

Water phase:
1. Weight of drug to be dissolved in RO water as per the formula
2. Preservative sodium benzoate 0.1%
3. Stabilizer citric acid 0.05%
4. Aqua = 8 liters
5. Sugar syrup 66.7% made by boiling in water, cool and filter, using to make emulsion palatable to taste

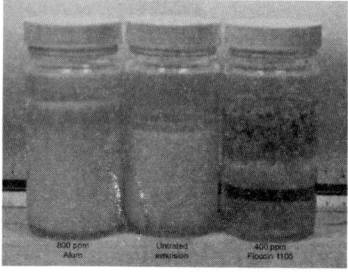

Emulsion

Method

Heat part A and part B separately at 60°C. Mix part A in part B slowly with constant emulsification for 10 minutes. Emulsion is ready and pack in 50 ml bottle. Yield must be greater than 97%.

Machine used

1. Bottle washing machine
2. Bottle drier machine
3. Stainless steel tank
4. Emulsifier
5. Volumetric filling machine

6. Capping machine
7. Batch printing machine
8. Label gumming machine
9. Taping and sealing cartons
10. Digital balance
11. Measuring cylinder

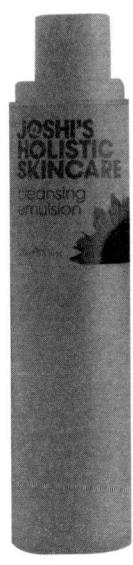

5 Multivitamins Nutritional Soft Capsule

Fundamental principles of multivitamin nutritional soft capsule formulation

Each soft gelatin capsule contains

Part A

Ingredients	Label claim	Overages%
1. Vitamin A (as palmitate)	1600 IU	35%
2. Vitamin D3	100 IU	27%
3. Vitamin B1	1 mg	10%
4. Vitamin B2	1 mg	10%
5. Vitamin B6	0.5 mg	10%
6. Vitamin B12	0.5 mcg	15%
7. Vitamin C	25 mg	10%
8. Vitamin E as acetate	5 mg	10%
9. Nicotinamide	15 mg	10%
10. Calcium pantothenate	1 mg	15%
11. Folic acid	50 mcg	10%
12. Calcium (as dicalcium phosphate)	75 mg	10%
13. Phosphorus (from DCP)	58 mg	10%
14. Copper (from copper sulphate)	50 mcg	10%
15. Iodine (from potassium iodide)	0.0075 mg	10%
16. Magnesium (as magnesium sulphate)	3 mg	10%
17. Manganese (as manganese sulphate)	0.5 mg	10%
18. Zinc (from zinc sulphate)	0.5 mg	10%
19. Potassium (from potassium sulphate)	2 mg	10%

Part B

Excipients:

1. Emulsifying agent soya bean oil 5%
2. Emulsifying agent hydrogenated vegetable oil 5%
3. Permitted colour orange 0.05%
4. Stabilizer citric acid 0.05%
5. Preservative sodium benzoate 0.1%
6. Antioxidant disodium EDTA 0.05%

Method

In part B, part A is mixed and all ingredients are dissolved in emulsifying agents. The dissolved ingredients are filled in soft gelatin capsule by machine. Heated filled gelatin capsule are shaped, cooled and cut to give form of filled soft gelatin capsule. Soft gelatin capsule are packed in blister pack or bottles with absorbent as silica granules and labeled. Yield % must be greater than 97%.

Machines used

1. Digital balance
2. Measuring cylinder
3. Capsule filling and sealing machine
4. Capsule disintegration
5. Capsule dissolution machine
6. Strip or blister machine
7. Batch printing machine
8. Label gumming machine
9. Taping and sealing cartons.

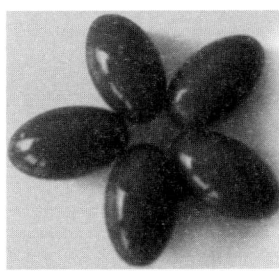

Soft capsules

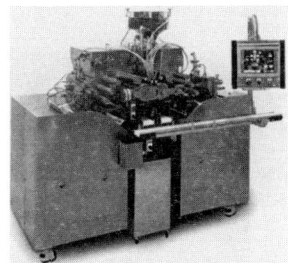

Soft capsule filling and sealing machine

Fundamental principles of strong solution formulation

Formula

1. *Sugar:* 3 teaspoonful in 50 ml of reverse osmosis water
2. Sodium chloride: ¼ teaspoonful in 50 ml of RO water
3. *Sodium benzoate:* 0.1% w/w
4. *Citric acid:* 0.1% w/w

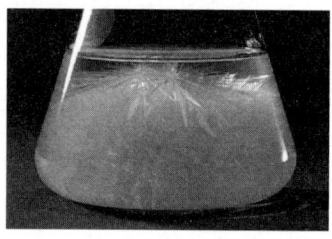

Strong solution

Method: Boil 1, 2, 3 and 4 to get strong solution. Filter the strong solution and cool the solution.

Uses: Laxative, antacid, nutritional supplement, counter irritant.

Doses: 100 ml

Dosage: 100 ml SOS

Storage: Store in cool place only.

Machine used

1. Stainless steel container of 100 litres volume
2. Heater or LPG gas and stove
3. Filters
4. Stirrer
5. Bottle washing machine

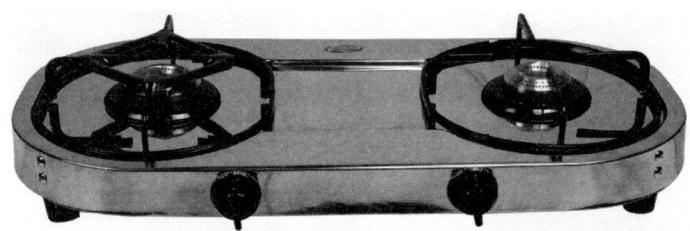

LPG stove

6. Bottle drier
7. Volumetric liquid filling machine
8. Capping machine
9. Batch printing machine
10. Label gumming machine
11. Taping and sealing cartons
12. Digital balance
13. Measuring cylinder.

7   *Liquid Syrup Technology*

Fundamental principles of liquid syrup

1. Weight of drug
2. Sweetening agent sugar syrup (66.7 grams of sugar in 100 ml of boiling water) or sorbitol 70% v/v syrup mix to sweet in taste
3. Solubising agent polyethylene glycol 0.05%
4. Thickening agent sodium CMC high viscosity 0.05%
5. Colouring agent tartrazine (yellow) (0.02% w/w)
6. Flavouring agent raspberry 0.5%
7. Preservative, methylparaben 0.08% w/w and propyl-paraben 0.04% w/w
8. Stabilizer, citric acid 0.05% w/w
9. Reverse osmosis water in volume equivalent the formula of product.

Method

Make sugar syrup in boiling water, cool and filter. Mix and stir 1, 2, 3, 4, 5, 6, 7, 8 and 9 for 15 minutes.

Liquid syrup is ready for packing in 50 ml, 100 ml plastic bottles. Yield must be greater than 99%.

Machines used

1. Digital balance
2. Measuring cylinder
3. Heater
4. Stainless steel bowl
5. Filter
6. Stirrer
7. Stainless steel tank
8. Volumetric filling machine

9. Capping machine
10. Batch printing machine
11. Label gumming machine
12. Taping and sealing cartons

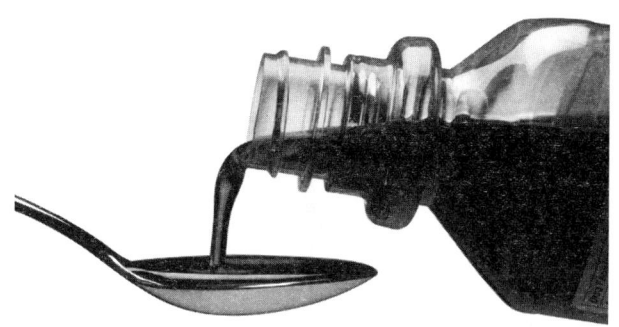

Cough syrup

8   *Pharmacy Calculations*

Metric system/practical calculation
Solids (weight)

State	Unit	Conversion
Powers, granules	Kilogram (kg)	1 ,000 grams
Tablets, capsules	Gram (g)	1,000 milligrams
	Milligram (mg)	1,000 micrograms (mcg)
	Microgram (mcg)	10^{-6} or $1/1000000$ g
	Nanogram (ncg)	10^{-9} or $1/1000000000$ g
	Picagram (pcg)	10^{-12} or $1/100000000000$ g
	Femtogram (fcg)	10^{-15} or $1/1000000000000000$ g
	Attogram (acg)	10^{-18} or $1/1000000000000000000$ g
	1 kilogram	2.20 pound avoirdupois (lb)

1 pound avoirdupois = 454 gm
1 ounce avoirdupois (oz) = 28.4 gm
1 ounce apothecary = 31.1 gm
1 pound apothecary (lb) = 373 gm
1 gram = 15.4 gr
1 grain (gr) = 64.8 milligrams

Gross weight = Weight of product + weight of packing
Tare weight   = Weight of packing
Net weight   = Weight of product
Net weight   = Gross weight – Tare weight

Liquids (Volume)

Water, alcohols	Litre (L)	= 1,000 millilitres (ml)
Oils	Millilitre (ml)	= 1,000 microlitres (mcl)

Microlitres (mcl) $= 10^{-6}$ or $1/1000000$ L
Nanolitre (ncl) $= 10^{-9}$ or $1/1000000000$ L
Picalitre (pcl) $= 10^{-12}$ or
  $1/1000000000000$ L
Femtogram (fcl) $= 10^{-15}$ or
  $1/1000000000000000$ L
Attolitre (acl) $= 10^{-18}$ or $1/$
  1000000000000000000 L

1 drop	=	0.06 ml
1 teaspoonful	=	5 ml
1 dessert spoonful	=	10 ml
1 tablespoonful	=	15 ml
1 wine glassful	=	60 ml
1 tea cupful	=	120 ml
1 tumblerful	=	240 ml
1 milliliter	=	16.2 minims
1 fluidounce	=	29.6 ml
1 pint	=	473 ml
1 gallon	=	3790 ml

International Unit (IU)
Vitamin A 1 mg = 2,907 IU of vitamin A acetate
Vitamin E synthetic 1 mg = 1.0 IU of d–alpha tocopheryl acetate
Vitamin E natural 1 mg = 1.49 IU of d–alpha tocopherol
Vitamin D 1 mg = 40,000 IU of vitamin D (D2 or D3)
Beta carotene 1 mg = 1,667 IU of beta carotene

Ratio Calculation
Lactose: Sucrose = 100:1, i.e. Lactose weight is 100 times more than sucrose weight.

Density = Weight/volume

Alcohol Dilution = Converting stronger alcohol to weaker alcohol is
Volume of stronger alcohol to be used = Volume needed * percentage needed/percentage used

Proof Spirit

Multiply the percentage strength of alcohol by 1.753 and deduct 100 from the product. If the result is positive it is known as over proof and if the result is negative then it is known as under proof.

The figure 1.753 is obtained as follows:

57.1 volume of ethyl alcohol = 100 volumes of proof spirit

1 volume of ethyl alcohol = 100/57.1 = 1.753 volumes of proof spirit.

Q.1. Find the strength of 90% v/v alcohol in terms of proof spirit?

Ans. 90 volumes of ethyl alcohol = 90*1.753–100

$$= 157.77–100$$
$$= + 57.77 \text{ or } 57.77° \text{ OP}$$

Q.2. Calculate the real strength of 40°OP and 50°UP?

Ans. *Applying the formula:*

40 Overproof means 100 + 40 = 140

Alcohol strength = 140/1.753 = 79.86% v/v

50 Underproof means 100–50 = 50

Alcohol strength = 50/1.753   = 28.52% v/v

Checking in OP and UP:

a. 79.86 * 1.753–100 = 139.99–100 = + 39.99 or 39.99 overproof (OP)

b. 28.52* 1.753–100 = 49.99–100 = –50.01 or 50.01 underproof (UP)

Weight by Volume

1% w/v = 1 gram of little amount solid (solute) dissolve in 100 ml of bigger amount liquid (solvent). Total volume is 100 ml.

Weight by Weight

1% W/W = 1 gram of little amount of solid (solute) mixed per 100 grams of bigger amount solid (solvent). Total weight is 100 grams.

Volume by Volume

1% V/V = 1 gram of little amount of liquid (solute) dissolve to make final volume equivalent to 100 ml of bigger amount of liquid. Total volume is 100 ml.

Parts Per Million (ppm)

2 ppm in 240 ml = 2/1000000 *240 ml = 0.00048 gm in 240 ml

Metric Linear Measure (Length, width, height, and thickness)

1 nanometer (nm)	=	10^{-9} m
1 micrometer (mcm)	=	10^{-6} m
1 millimeter (mm)	=	10^{-3} m
1 centimeter (cm)	=	10^{-2} m
1 decimeter (dm)	=	10^{-1} m
1 meter (m)	=	1.0 m
1 kilometer (km)	=	1000.0 m
1 meter	=	39.4 inches
1 inch	=	2.54 cm = 25.4 mm
1 micrometer	=	1/1000 mm = 10^{-6} m
	=	1/25,400 inch

Temperature

The relationship between Centigrade (C) and Fahrenheit (F) degrees is 9 (°C) = 5 (°F) – 160

Milliequivalents

Molecular weight	=	mg/mmol (millimol)
mEq (milliequivalent)	=	mmol/valence

Power

1 kilowatts (KW)	=	1.3410 Horsepower (HP)
1 kilowatt	=	1,000 watts (W)
1 Horsepower	=	746 watts
1 BTU (British thermal unit)	=	1055 joules
1 Horsepower-hour	=	2684520 joules
1 kilowatt-hour	=	3600000 joules
1 watt hour	=	600 joules

Area

1 karam	=	5.5 feet
1 marla	=	9 square karmas
20 marlas	=	1 kanal
160 marlas	=	1 acre
1 kanal	=	1/8 acre
100 acres	=	1 hectare
100 hectare	=	1 square kilometer
144 square inches	=	1 square foot
12 inches	=	1 foot
43560 square feet	=	1 acre
640 acres	=	1 square mile

Suspension Technology

Fundamental principles of suspension formulation

1. Weight of drug
2. Sodium CMC 0.5% w/w (suspending agent)
3. Glycerin 0.05% v/v (wetting agent)
4. Sodium chloride 0.02% w/w (flocculating agent)
5. Methylparaben 0.08% w/w and propylparaben 0.04% w/w (preservative)
6. Tartrazine (yellow) 0.02% w/w (colouring agent)
7. Sugar syrup 66.7% w/v q.s. (sweetening agent)
8. Raspberry 0.21% w/w (flavouring agent)
9. RO water q.s.

Method

Mix and stir 1, 9, and 2, 3, 4, 5, 6, 7, 8 for 15 minutes in colloidal mill. After chemical test approval, suspension is ready for packing in 50 ml, 100 ml plastic bottles. Yield must be greater than 97%.

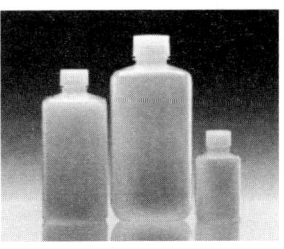

Suspension bottle

Machines used

1. Bottle washing machine
2. Bottle drier machine
3. Stainless steel tank
4. Volumetric liquid filling machine
5. Capping machine
6. Batch printing machine
7. Label gumming machine
8. Taping and sealing cartons
9. Digital balance
10. Measuring cylinder

10 Antibiotic Dry Syrup Technology

Fundamental principles of antibiotic dry syrup

Part A (Drug part)

1. Weight of drug
2. Sweetening agent sugar milled 97% w/w
3. Binding agent sodium carboxy methylcellulose 1% w/w in 50% v/v, ethanol and 50% v/v RO water

   Mix 1, 2, and 3 and make dry granules

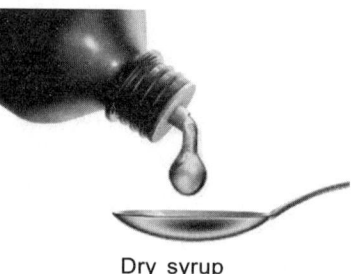
Dry syrup

Part B (Pharmaceautical excipient part)

4. Sugar milled 97% w/w
5. Binding agent sodium carboxycellulose 1% w/w in RO water
6. Buffering agent acidic citric acid to adjust pH= 6.00
7. Preservatives methylparaben (0.08%w/w), propylparaben (0.04% w/w)
8. Flavouring agent raspberry 0.21% w/w
9. Colour agent erythrosine HD 0.02% w/w

   Mix, 5, 6, 7, 8, 9 and 4 and make dry granules

Method

Dry mix part A and part B in such a way that weight of drug and excipients must be equivalent in the final volume making and weight of drug.

Dry syrup is ready for packing in 30 ml, 60 ml plastic bottles. Yield % must be greater than 93%.

Machines used

1. Mass mixer
2. Hot air drier
3. Oscillating granulator
4. Multi mill
5. Drum mixer
6. Bottle washing machine
7. Bottle drier
8. Capping machine
9. Batch printing machine
10. Label gumming machine
11. Taping and sealing cartons
12. Digital balance
13. Measuring cylinder

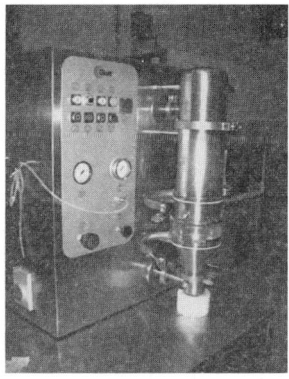

Fluid bed drier

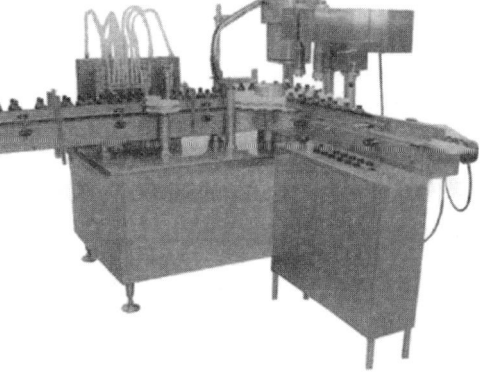

Automatic filling and sealing maching

Fundamental principles of hard capsule formulation

1. Weight of drug and weight of excipients (in metric system)
2. Dry mixing (mixing drug with absorbent magnesium carbonate 0.1% w/w, filler, glidant, starch 0.5% w/w, antiadhesive magnesium stearate 0.2% if needed, anti dusting vitamin E vegetable oil 0.5% w/v)
3. Capsulation (to make finished capsules)
4. Packing (Strip, blister, alu, 15 kg HMHDPE drums)

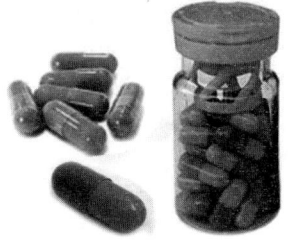

Bottle pack of hard capsules

Quality control and quality assurance for 20 capsules is
*Weight variation = Weight of capsule ± 5%
*Thickness = Size of capsule ± 5%
*Hardness = No capsule breaking

Clean capsules: No powder on capsules

Rate of disintegration: At 37 ± 5°C capsules (within 30 minutes) must disintegrate the powders and pass through the sieve.

Dissolution test: 100% capsule must dissolve and weight of drug must be equivalent to the label claim by chemical analysis within 1 hour.

Storage: Airtight packing with bag of silica.

Shell size	Approximately weight of acetyl salicylic acid
000	1 gram
00	650 milligrams
0	500 milligrams
1	320 milligrams

2	250 milligrams
3	200 milligrams
4	150 milligrams
5	10 milligrams

Yield % must be greater than 97%.

Machines used

1. Double cone blender
2. Capsule filling machine
3. Capsule disintegration
4. Capsule dissolution machine
5. Strip machine or blister machine
6. Taping and sealing cartons
7. Digital balance.

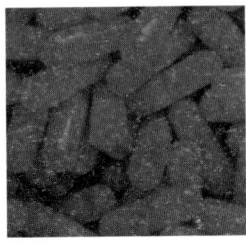

Coloured gelatin
capsule red/red, size 3

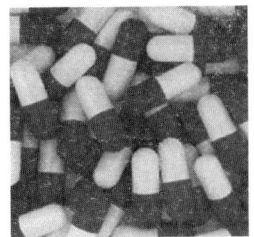

Gelatin capsule
red/ white, size 00

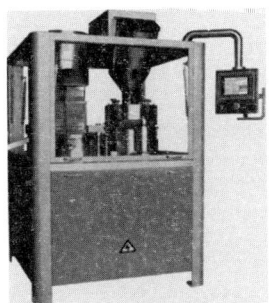

Automatic capsule filling machine

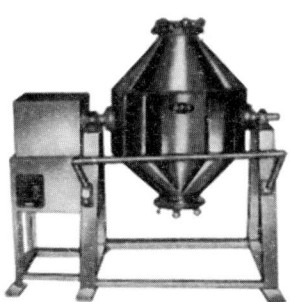

Double cone blender

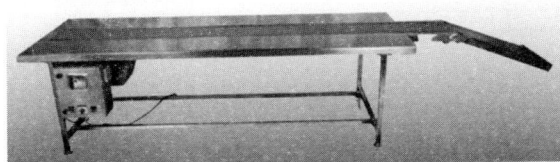

Packing conveyor

Fundamental principles of dry injection formulation

1. Weight of drug
2. Blending in sterile area if two or more drugs are weighed
3. No excipients
4. Weighing, filling, rubbering and sealing in vials

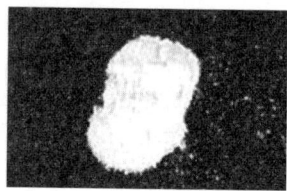

Dry powder

After chemical test, sterility test, pyrogen test, leak test, vials are ready for packing. Yield % must be greater than 97%

Machines used

1. Vial washing machine
2. Vial drier machine
3. Laminar flow machine
4. Vial filling, plugging and sealing machine
5. Label gumming machine
6. Batch printing machine
7. Taping and sealing cartons
8. 20 litres tank containing formaldehyde and potassium permanganate for fumigation.
9. Digital balance.

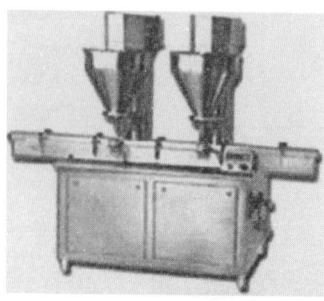

Vial filling machine

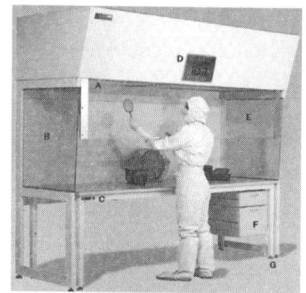

Laminar air flow

13 Fluid Juice Technology

Fundamental principles of fluid juice formulation

1. Sweetening agent sugar syrup 66.7 % w/v in boiling water or sorbitol syrup 70% v/v
2. One synthetic flavouring agent 0.21% w/w like apple, carrot, orange, mango, lemon.
3. Preservatives methylparaben 0.08% w/w, propylparaben 0.04% w/w
4. Vechile RO water quantity sufficient to produce synthetic flavouring taste
5. Stablizer sodium EDTA 0.02% w/w
6. Sodium lauryl sulphate 0.01% w/w
7. Buffering agent acidic citric acid 0.02% w/w

Method

Dissolve 1, 2, 3, 4, 5, 6 and 7. Pack in glass bottles, plastic bottles, tetra pack. Yield % must be greater than 99%.

Machine used

1. Bottle washing machine
2. Bottle drier
3. Stainless steel tank
4. LPG gas and stove
5. Stirrer
6. Filter press
7. Volumetric liquid filling machine
8. Capping machine
9. Batch printing machine
10. Label gumming machine
11. Taping and sealing cartons
12. Digital balance
13. Measuring cylinder

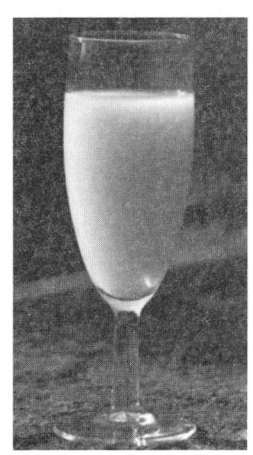

Fluid juice

14 Analgesic Gel Formulation

Fundamental principles of analgesic gel formulation
1. Weight of analgesic drug like nimesulide, etc.
2. Gelling agent carbopol 0.66%
3. Stabilizer disodium EDTA 0.1%
4. Preservative sodium benzoate 0.1%
5. Binder polyvinylpyrrolidone 0.05%
6. Humectant glycerin 1%
7. Colourant green 0.1%
8. Gelling agent aloe vera gel 0.5%
9. Perfume lavender oil 0.5%
10. RO water quantity sufficient to make 100%.

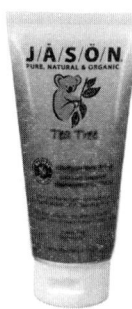

Gel

Method
Dissolve 1 to 9 and then dissolve 2 in the end and pack in 30 gm tubes. Yield must be greater than 97%.

Machines used
1. Digital balance
2. Measuring cylinder
3. Stainless steel tank
4. Stirrer
5. Gel filling machine
6. Batch printing machine
7. Label gumming machine
8. Taping and sealing cartons.

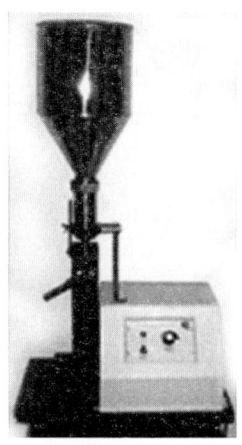

Gel filling machine

15   *Dusting Powder Technology*

Fundamental principles of dusting powder formulation
1. Weight of drugs for example = 25%
2. Weight of starch powder = 75%

Method
Mix 1 and 2 in mass mixer for 15 minutes, transfer and pack in 50 gm bottle. Yield must be greater than 97%.

Machine used
1. Digital balance
2. Drum mixer
3. Powder filling machine
4. Batch printing machine
5. Label gumming machine
6. Taping and sealing cartons
7. Digital balance

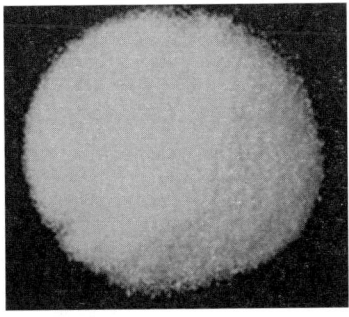

Dusting powder technology

16 Ointment Formulation Technology

Fundamental principles of ointment formulation
1. Emollient polyethylene glycol 400 = 1 liter
2. Emulsifying wax polyethylene glycol 4000 = 1 kg
3. Preservative sodium benzoate 0.1% = 2 grams
4. Stabilizer disodium EDTA 0.05% = 1 gram
5. Povidone-iodine 5% = 100 grams

Method
Heat 1, 2 at 60°C. Mix with emulsifier rotating. Add 3, 4, and 5 and emulsify for 10 minutes. Ointment is made. Transfer in small packing 15 gm using filling machine with heater. Yield must be greater than 97%.

Machines used
1. Planetary mixer
2. Triple roll mill
3. Manual/automatic tube filling machine
4. Tube sealing machine
5. Batch printing machine
6. Gumming machine
7. Taping and sealing cartons
8. Digital balance
9. Measuring cylinder

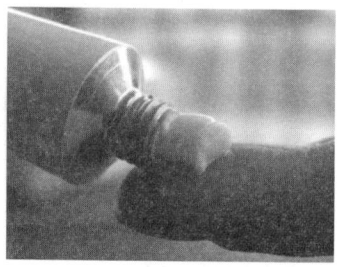

Ointment

Liquid Parenterals Technology

Fundamental principles of liquid parenterals (infusion, ampoule, vial) formulation

1. Weight of drug
2. Distilled water (vehicle)
3. Sodium EDTA 0.05% w/w (stabiliser)
4. Citric acid to control the pH in acidic (buffering agent)
5. Sodium chloride 0.9% w/w (tonicity)
6. Methylparaben 0.08% w/w, propylparaben 0.04% w/w (preservatives)

Mix and stir 1, 2, 3, 4, 5, 6 in small volume. Then stir the solution in required volume for 1 hour.

Ampoule, vial and infusion is ready for packing after chemical test, sterility test, and leak test passes approval. Yield% must be greater than 99%.

Machine used

1. Ampoule, vial, infusion washing machine
2. Ampoule, vial, infusion drier machine
3. Stainless steel tank
4. Stirrer
5. Filter press
6. Laminar flow machine
7. Volumetric liquid filling machine
8. Capping machine
9. Autoclave
10. Batch printing machine
11. Label gumming machine
12. Taping and sealing carton

13. For fumigation 20 litres small tank containing formaldehyde and potassium permanganate.
14. Digital balance
15. Measuring cylinder

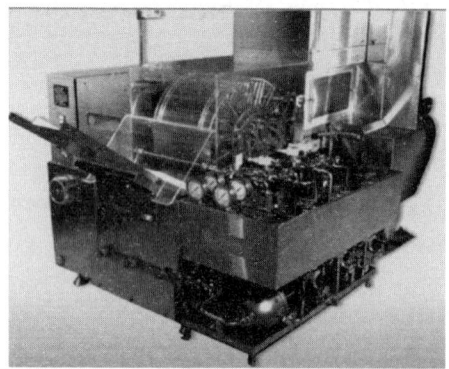

Ampoule washing machine

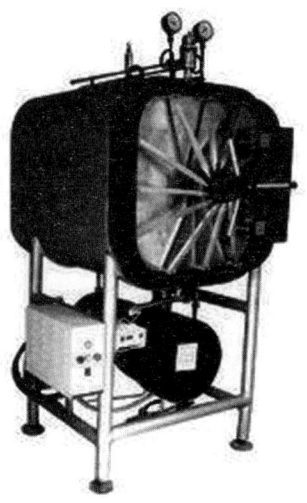

Rectangular autoclave working
at 121° for 15 minutes

Fundamental principles of herbal powder making

1. Sorting of dry leaves from small wood sticks.
2. Dry leaves are grinding in (pulverizer) grinding machine
3. Grinded material are passed through sieve to obtain 200 mesh size particles

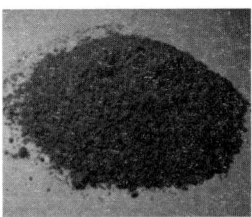

Herbal powder

After test approval, 25 kg, 50 kg packing (polythene bags, LDPE bags) are sealed. Yield % must be greater than 25%.

Machines used

1. Grinder machine
2. Digital balance
3. Powder filling machine

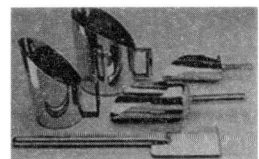

Stainless steel scoops

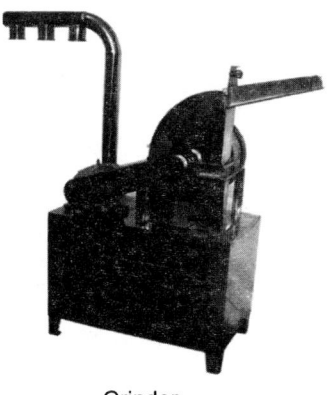

Grinder

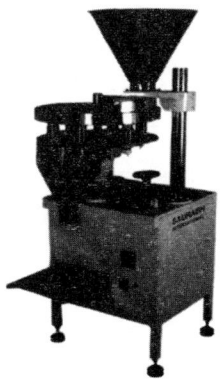

Powder filling machine

Fundamental principles of liquid extract formulation

1. Weight of herbs
2. Cleaning of herbs 2 times with water to remove dust, particles, soil, etc.
3. Cutting of herbs in smaller pieces for uniform distribution
4. Soaking the herbs in cool water for at least 12 hours to make herb soft, hence low value of manufacturing
5. Heating the soaked herbs in RO water for 3 to 6 hours for 60 litres volume so that drug is extracted in water
6. Filtering the hot liquid extract
7. Cooling the liquid extract for 12 hours
8. Adding preservatives methylparaben 0.08% w/v and propyl paraben 0.04% w/v and stir for 10 minutes
9. Packing in 35 litres HMHDPE Jerry Canes or 100 ml bottles. Yield % must be greater than 70%.

Machine used

1. Stainless steel container of 100 litres volume
2. Heater or LPG gas and stove
3. Filters
4. Stirrer
5. Bottle washing machine
6. Bottle drier
7. Volumetric liquid filling machine
8. Capping machine
9. Batch printing machine
10. Label gumming machine
11. Taping and sealing cartons
12. Digital balance
13. Measuring cylinder.

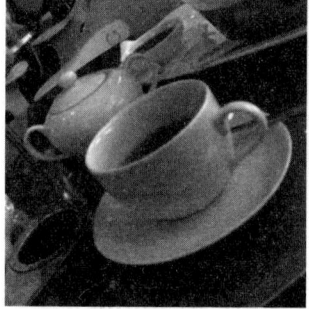

Liquid extract

Tincture Technology

Fundamental principles of tincture formulation

1. 2 times cleaning of small pieces of fresh drug with clean water
2. Weight of fresh drug in metric system
3. Volume of ethanol like 25% v/v, 40% v/v, 50% v/v
4. Soaking of fresh drug in ethanol for 7 days (maceration) in wooden drums
5. Filtration of drug dissolved in ethanol
6. Sodium benzoate 0.05% w/v .... preservative
7. Airtight packing in glass or plastic bottles. Yield must be greater than 97%

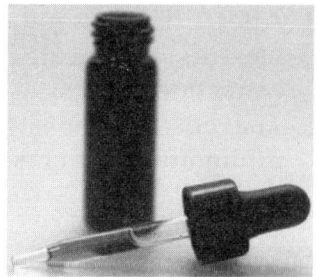

Tincture bottle

Machines used

1. Grinder machine to make small pieces
2. Digital balance
3. Measuring cylinder
4. Filter
5. Stirrer
6. Stainless steel tank
7. Volumetric tincture filling machine
8. Capping machine
9. Batch printing machine
10. Label gumming machine
11. Taping and sealing cartons.

Fundamental principles of essential oil manufacturing

1. Small pieces of fresh plant is cleaned with water 2 times
2. Cleaned small pieces of fresh plant 1 part and RO water 2 parts is added in oil extraction plant
3. Oil extraction plant is closed with nuts and bolts and oil extraction is kept at 60°C (steam distillation)
4. After 1 hour essential oil is produced (by condensation of vapours) and heated RO water keep on circulating in the extraction plant
5. The process is repeated for next batch. Essential oil is packed in aluminum container, 10 ml bottles. Yield % must be greater than 0.4%.

Machine used

1. Oil extraction machine
2. Volumetric filling machine
3. Batch printing machine
4. Label gumming machine
5. Taping and sealing cartons
6. Digital balance
7. Measuring cylinder

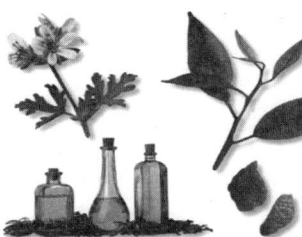

Essential oil

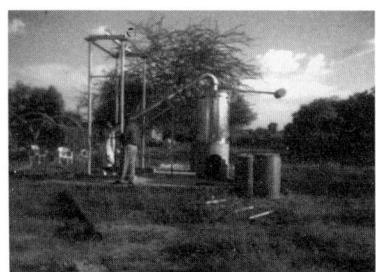

Essential oil distillation

Fundamental principles of body spray/after shave formulation

1. Chlorhexidine diacetate antibacterial (soluble in alcohol and RO water) 0.15% w/w
2. Phenyl ethyl alcohol perfume 95 ml
3. RO water 5 ml
4. Methylparaben 0.08% w/w, propylparaben 0.04% w/w

Method

Dissolve 1, 2, 3 and 4 and pack in 50 ml, 100 ml spray bottles. Yield % must be greater than 99%.

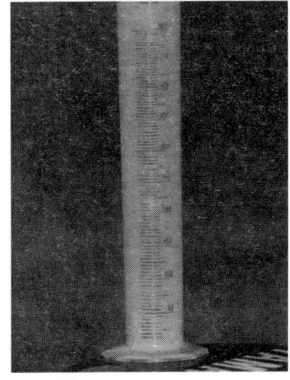

Body spray

Machines used

1. Bottle washing machine
2. Bottle drier machine
3. Stainless steel tank
4. Stirrer

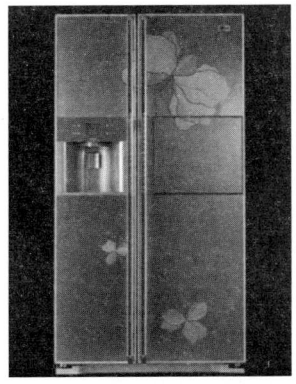

Glass bottle drier

Measuring cylinder

5. Volumetric liquid filling machine
6. Capping machine
7. Label gumming machine
8. Tapping and sealing carton
9. Digital balance
10. Measuring cylinder.

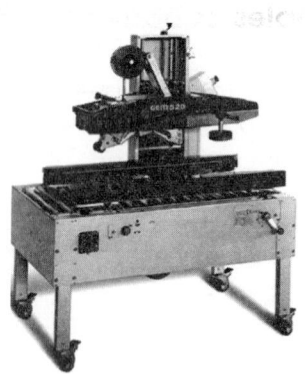

Tapping machine

23   *Cream Technology*

Fundamental principles of cream formulation

1. *Water phase*
   a. Vehicle RO water = 8 litres
   b. Sunscreen agent PABA = 0.03% w/w = 3 grams
   c. Preservatives methylparaben = 0.08% w/w (8 grams), propylparaben = 0.04% w/w (4 grams)
   d. White colour to skin hydroquinone 1% w/w = 100 grams
   e. Essence lavender oil = 50 ml

2. *Oil phase*
   a. Emollient mineral oil = 1 litre
   b. Emollient emulsifying wax = 1 kg

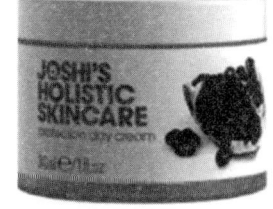

Cream

Method

Dissolve in water phase a, b, c, d. Boil/melt at 60°C water phase and oil phase separately. Now slowly mix oil phase in water phase at 60°C in emulsifier for 15 minutes. Mix lavender oil and emulsify for 5 minutes. Cream is ready for packing in tubes. Yield % must be greater than 97%.

Machines used

1. Stainless steel tank
2. Emulsifier
3. Heater
4. Cream filling machine
5. Batch printing machine
6. Label gumming machine
7. Taping and sealing machine
8. Digital balance
9. Measuring cylinder

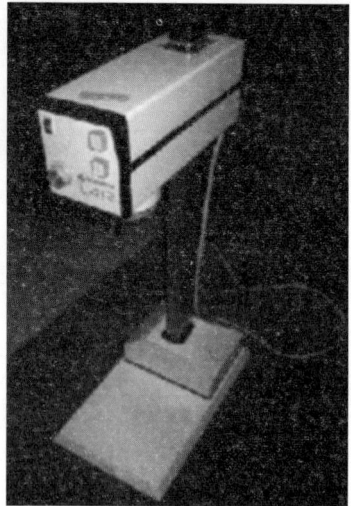

Emulsifier

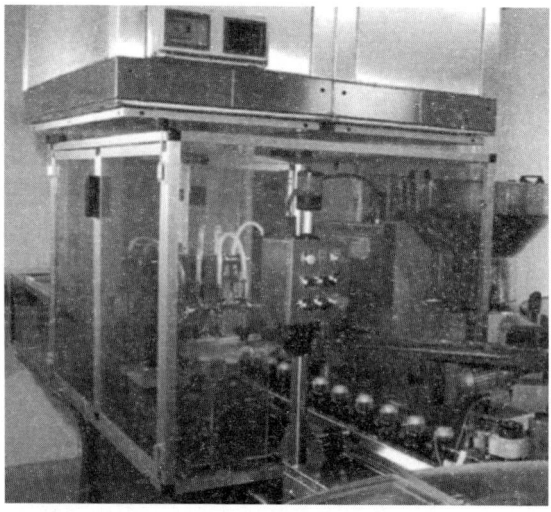

Filling machine

Fundamental principles of shaving cream formulation

Formula: Weight by weight

Part A
1. Emulsifier palmic acid = 9.5%
2. Emulsifier stearic acid = 7.5%
3. Humectant glycerin = 23.50%
4. Perfume lavender oil= 0.5%
5. Preservative sodium benzoate= 0.1%
   Total part A% = 41.10%

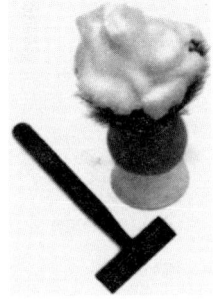

Shaving cream

Part B
1. Soft soap potassium hydroxide = 3% for shaving cream
2. Hard soap sodium hydroxide = 1%
3. Coconut oil = 32%
4. Olive oil = 20%
5. Aqua = 3%
   Total part B= 58.90%

Heat part A and part B separately at 60°C. Mix part A in part B slowly. Shaving cream is formed.

Olive oil, vitamin E oil, soya bean oil, vitamin A and K, cocoa butter for making soft shaving cream. Palm oil for making hard shaving cream.

Machines used
1. Digital balance
2. Measuring cylinder
3. Planetary mixer
4. Triple roll mill

5. Manual/semi/automatic tube filling machine
6. Tube sealing machine
7. Batch printing machine
8. Label gumming machine
9. Taping and sealing the cartons.

Fundamental principles of creamy soap bar (soft soap)

Formula: Weight by weight

Part A:

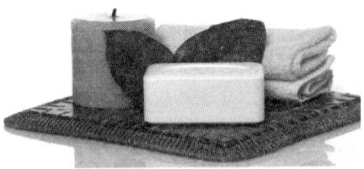

1. Emulsifier palmic acid = 9.5%
2. Emulsifier stearic acid = 7.5%
3. Humectant glycerin = 23.50%
4. Perfume lavender oil = 0.5%
5. Preservative sodium benzoate = 0.1%
   Total part A% = 41.10%

Soap bar

Part B:

1. Soft soap potassium hydroxide = 2.90%
2. Hard soap sodium hydroxide = 1%
3. Coconut oil = 32%
4. Olive oil = 20%
5. Aqua = 3%
   Total part B= 58.90%

   Heat part A and part B separately at 60°C. Mix part A in part B slowly. Creamy soap is formed.

   Olive oil, vitamin E oil, soya bean oil, vitamin A and K, cocoa butter for making soft soap. Palm oil for making hard soap.

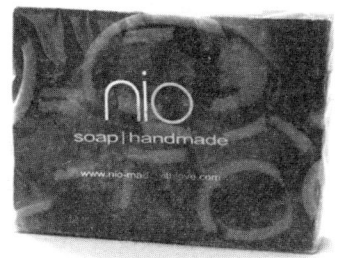

Transparent soap bar

   For transparent soap use sorbitol, PEG 400 and glycerin in place of palmic acid and stearic acid.

   For detergent cake detergent builder, detergent fillers and detergent fillers borax is mostly used in % and lesser % of oils, emulsifiers are used to reduce the cost.

   For soap powder has lesser % of aqua and granules of soap is made.

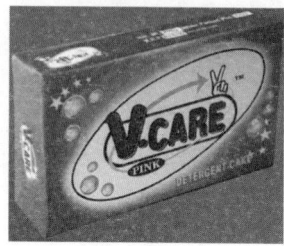

Detergent cake

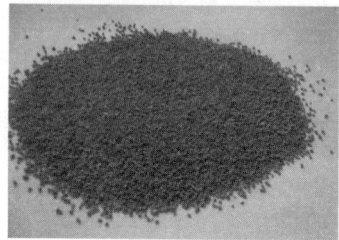

Detergent powder

Machines used

1. Soap making machine
2. Soap cutter machine
3. Soap wrapper machine
4. Soap noodle machine
5. Digital balance
6. Measuring cylinder

Toilet soap: 10 to 100 grams. Yield % must be greater than 92%.

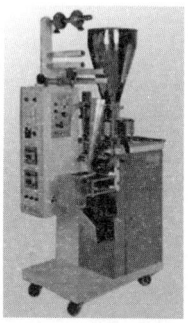

Soap making machine

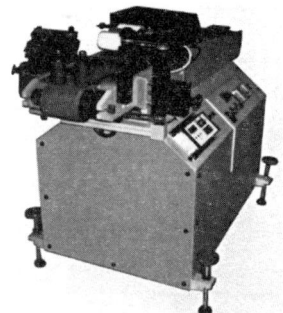

Soap, detergent cutter

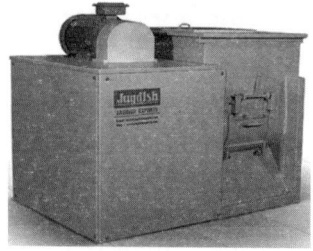

Soap noodle machine

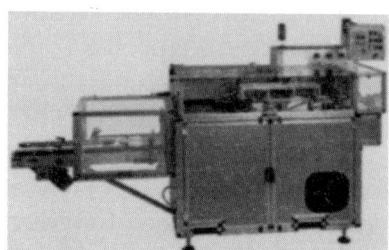

Soap wrapper machine

Fundamental principles of hair gel formulation
1. Gelling agent carbopol 0.66%
2. Stabilizer disodium EDTA 0.1%
3. Preservative sodium benzoate 0.1%
4. Binder polyvinylpyrrolidone 0.05%
5. Humectant glycerin 1%
6. Colourant green 0.1%
7. Gelling agent aloe vera gel 0.5%
8. Perfume rose water 10%
9. RO water quantity sufficient to make 100%.

Method
Dissolve 2 to 9 and then dissolve 1 and pack in 500 grams jars. Yield must be greater than 97%.

Machines used
1. Digital balance
2. Measuring cylinder
3. Stainless steel tank
4. Stirrer
5. Gel filling machine
6. Batch printing machine
7. Label gumming machine
8. Taping and sealing cartons.

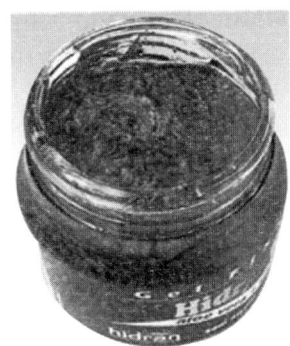

Hair gel

27   *Lotion Technology*

Fundamental principles of lotion formulation

1. *Water phase*
   a. Vehicle reverse osmosis water = 22 litres
   b. Sunscreen agent PABA = 0.03% w/w = 7.20 grams
   c. Preservatives methylparaben 0.08% w/w = 19.20 grams, propylparaben = 0.04% w/w = 9.60 grams
   d. Perfume lavender oil = 50 ml
2. *Oil phase*
   a. Emollient mineral oil = 1 litre
   b. Emollient emulsifying wax stearic acid = 1 kg

Method

Dissolve water phase a, b, c, d in container. Boil/melt at 60°C water phase and oil phase separately. Slowly mix oil phase in water phase at 60°C in emulsifier for 15 minutes. Mix lavender oil and emulsify for 5 minutes. Lotion is ready for packing in plastic bottles. Yield must be greater than 97%.

Machines used

1. Stainless steel tank
2. Emulsifier
3. Heater
4. Lotion filling machine
5. Batch printing machine
6. Label gumming machine
7. Taping and sealing machine
8. Digital balance
9. Measuring cylinder

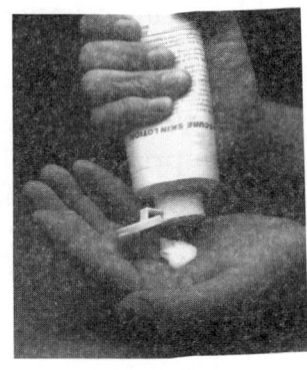

Skin lotion

28   *Shampoo Technology*

Fundamental principles of shampoo formulation

1. Detergent sodium lauryl sulphate (50 % v/v) = 100,000 ml
2. Detergent reetha (1% v/v) = 1000 ml
3. Detergent shekakai (1% v/v) = 1000 ml
4. Preservatives methyl paraben (0.08% w/w) = 160 grams, propylparaben (0.04% w/w) = 80 grams
5. Vehicle reverse osmosis water (48% v/v) = 96,000 ml
6. Thicker sodium chloride (2% w/w) = 400 grams
7. Essence oil (0.3% v/v): 60 ml

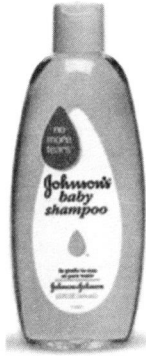

Shampoo bottle

Method

Mix and stir 1, 2, 3, 4, 5 and 6 for 15 minutes. Now add 7 and stir for 5 minutes.

Shampoo is ready for packing in sachets or plastic bottles 50 ml, 100 ml, 150 ml, 200 ml, 250 ml, 500 ml. Yield must be greater than 97%.

Machines used

1. Bottle washing machine
2. Stainless steel tank
3. Shampoo/sachets filling machine
4. Batch printing machine
5. Label gumming machine
6. Taping and sealing cartons
7. Digital balance
8. Measuring cylinder.

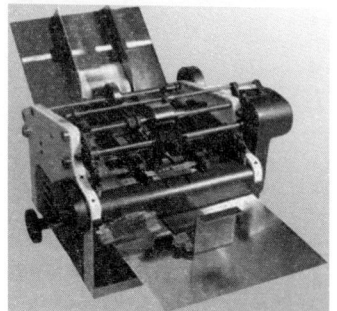

Batch printing machine

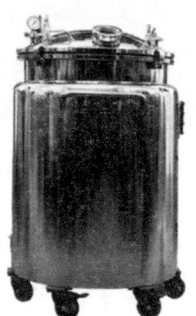

Stainless steel tank

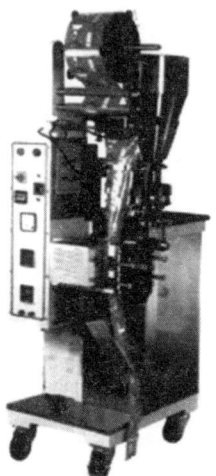

Batch printing machine

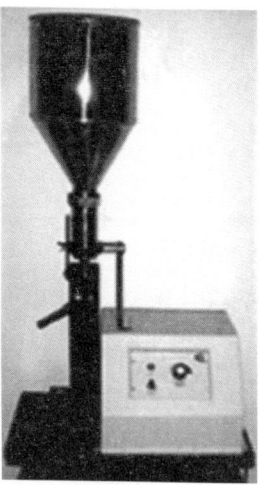

Shampoo filling machine

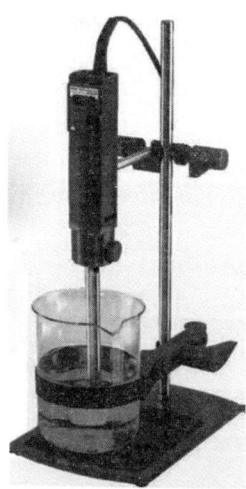

Stirrer quality ss 316

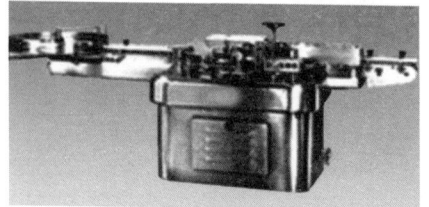

Bottle labelling machine

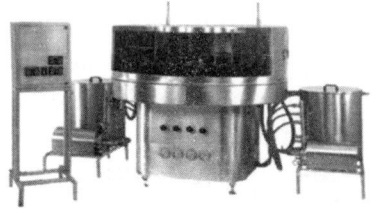

Bottle washing machine

Fundamental principles of toothpaste

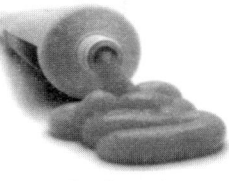

Toothpaste

1. Abrasive and polishing materials calcium phosphate 56% w/w
2. White agenting, anti plaque sodium fluoride 0.0243% w/w, sodium hydroxide 0.01% w/w
3. Detergents and foaming agent sodium lauryl phosphate 1% w/w
4. Humectant glycerin 22% w/v, sorbitol (sweeting agent) 16% w/v
5. Binding agent CMC 1 % w/w
6. Sweetening agent saccharine sodium 0.1% w/w
7. Flavour clove oil 1% v/v
8. Preservative methylparaben 0.08% w/w, propyl paraben 0.04% w/w
9. Colour blue (brilliant blue FCF) 0.02% w/w
10. Anticavity sodium bicarbonate 1% w/w
11. RO water sufficient to produce toothpaste

Method
Mix 5 in 10 then mix 1, 2, 3, 4, 6, 7, 8, 9, 10 and pack in plastic or aluminum tubes. Yield % must be greater than 97%.

Machines used
1. Stirrer
2. Toothpaste mixer (planetary mixer)
3. Triple roll mill
4. Toothpaste filling machine
5. Tooth sealing machine
6. Batch printing machine

7. Show box gumming machine
8. Tapping and sealing cartons
9. Digital balance

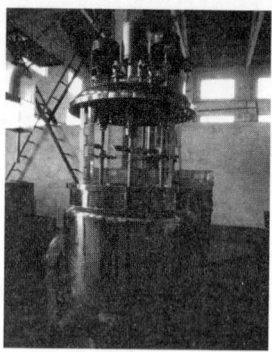

Planetary mixer

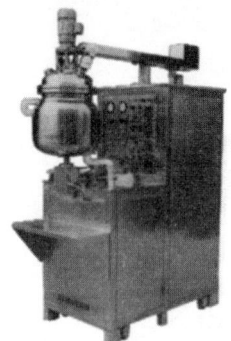

Filling machine

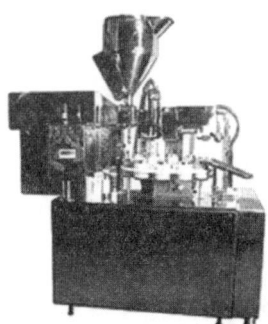

Semi automatic sealing machine

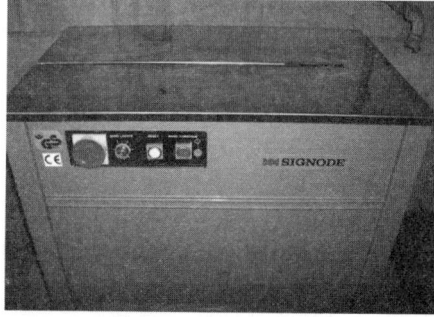

Strapping machine

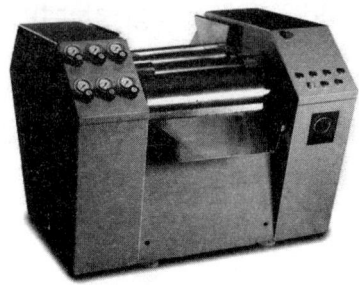

Triple roll mill

30   *Better Cream Formulation*

Fundamental principles of better cream formulation

1. Water phase
   a. Vehicle RO water = 8 litres
   b. Sunscreen agent PABA = 0.03% w/w = 3 grams
   c. Preservatives methylparaben = 0.08 % w/w (8 grams), propylparaben = 0.04% w/w (4 grams)
   d. White colour to skin hydroquinone 1% w/w =100 grams
   e. Essence lavender oil = 50 ml
   f. Emollient glycerin = 0.01% v/v (1 ml)
   g. Emollient triethanolamine = 0.01% v/v (1 ml)
   h. Antibacterial imidazolindinyl urea = 0.04% w/w (4 grams)
   i. Synergistic EDTA disodium = 0.02% w/w (2 grams)
   j. Thickner carbomer = 0.01% w/w (1 gram)
   k. Nutrient sodium lactate = 0.01% w/w (1 gram)
   l. Tincture glycyrrhiza = 0.01% v/v (1 ml)
   m. Antibacterial glabra = 0.01% w/w (1 gram)

2. Oil phase
   a. Emollient mineral oil = 950 ml
   b. Emollient tocopheryl acetate = 45 ml
   c. Propylene glycol = 5 ml
   d. Emollient emulsifying wax stearic acid= 975 grams
   e. Emollient emulsifying granules = 20 grams
   f. Emollient emulsifying wax glyceryl strearate = 5 grams

Method
Dissolve in water phase a, b, c, d, e, f, g, h, i, j, k, l, m. Boil/ melt at 60°C water phase and oil phase separately. Now slowly mix oil phase in water phase at 60°C in emulsifier for

15 minutes. Mix lavender oil and emulsify for 5 minutes. Cream is ready for packing in tubes. Yield % must be greater than 97%.

Machines used
1. Stainless steel tank
2. Emulsifier
3. Heater
4. Cream filling machine
5. Batch printing machine
6. Label gumming machine
7. Taping and sealing machine
8. Digital balance
9. Measuring cylinder

31   *Gum Paint Formulation*

Fundamental principles of gum paint astringent formulation

1. Astringent and antiseptic tannic acid 2% w/v
2. Astringent zinc chloride 1% w/v
3. Antibacterial cetrimide 0.1%
4. Vehicle glycerin 96.9% v/v

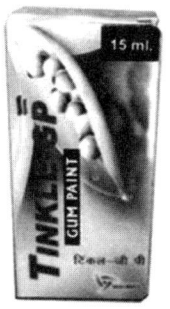 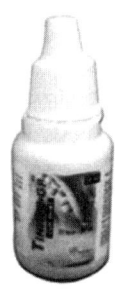

Gum paint

Method

Dissolve 1, 2, and 3 in 4 and stir the solution for 15 minutes. Yield % not less than 95%.

Machines used

1. Bottle washing machine
2. Bottle drier machine
3. Stainless steel tank
4. Stirrer
5. Volumetric liquid filling machine
6. Capping machine
7. Batch printing machine
8. Label gumming machine
9. Taping and sealing cartons
10. Digital balance
11. Measuring cylinder

Hair Oil
32 *Formulation Technology*

Fundamental principles of hair oil formulation
1. Amla or almond oil 1%
2. Mineral oil liquid paraffin 98.5%
3. Colorant green 0.1 %
4. Preservative sodium benzoate 0.1 %
5. Perfume lavender oil 0.5%

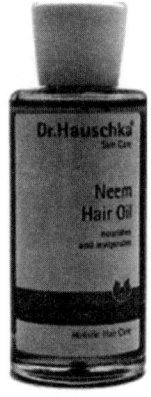

Method
Mix and stir 1 to 5 and pack in 100 ml bottle.
Yield must be greater than 99%

Machines Used
  1. Bottle washing machine

Hair oil

  2. Bottle drier machine
  3. Stainless steel tank
  4. Volumetric oil filling machine
  5. Capping
  6. Batch printing machine
  7. Label gumming machine
  8. Taping and sealing cartons
  9. Digital balance
10. Measuring cylinder

33 Mouth Wash and Gargle Technology

Fundamental principles of mouth wash and gargle
1. Vehicle RO water 50% v/v
2. Antibacterial hydrogen peroxide (3% v/v) 50% v/v
3. Preservatives methylparaben 0.08% w/w, propylparaben 0.04% w/w

Method
Dissolve and stir 1, 2 an 3 and pack in glass or plastic bottles. Yield must be greater than 99%

Machines used
1. Bottle washing machine
2. Bottle drier machine
3. Stainless steel tank
4. Stirrer
5. Volumetric liquid filling machine
6. Capping machine
7. Batch printing machine
8. Label gumming machine
9. Taping and sealing cartons
10. Digital balance
11. Measuring cylinder.

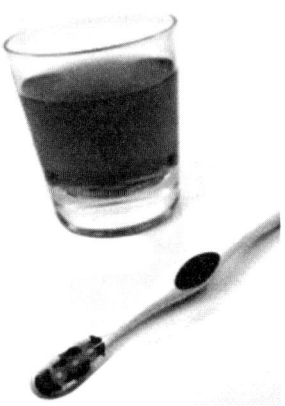

Mouth wash, gargle and brush

Fundamental principles of shaving gel formulation
1. Detergent sodium lauryl sulphate 75% v/v
2. Vehicle RO water 24.47% v/v
3. Thickener sodium chloride 2% w/w
4. Preservative methylparaben 0.08% w/w and propylparaben 0.04%w/w
5. Menthol oil 0.5% v/v
6. Colour blue (brilliant blue FCF) 0.21% w/w
7. Essence lavender oil 0.03% v/v

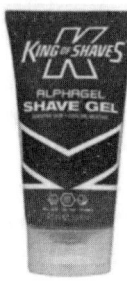

Shaving gel

Method
Dissolve 5 in 1, then dissolve 2, 4, 3, 6 and 7 and pack in 50 ml, 100 ml and 200 ml plastic tubes. Yield must be greater than 97%.

Machines used
1. Stainless steel tank
2. Stirrer
3. Gel filling machine
4. Batch printing machine
5. Label gumming machine
6. Taping and sealing machine
7. Digital balance
8. Measuring cylinder

35 Lip Gloss Formulation

Fundamental principles of formulation of lip gloss, FDA approved

Oils

Lip gloss

1. Minerals oil—95%
2. Castor oil—2%
3. Olive oil—0.5%
4. Peanut oil—0.5%
5. Mustard oil—0.5%
6. Menthol oil (cooling effect)—0.5%
7. Aroma oil (perfume)—0.5%
8. Vitamin A oil (antioxidant)—0.25%
9. Vitamin E oil (antioxidant)—0.25%
10. BHA (butylated hydroxyanisole as preservative for oils)—0.02% or 200 parts per million (ppm)
11. Colours—green, orange, blue–0.05% each

Method

Dissolve and stir 1 to 11 and pack in 10 ml glass or plastic bottles. Yield must be greater than 97%.

Machines used

1. Bottle washing machine
2. Bottle drier machine
3. Stainless steel tank
4. Stirrer
5. Volumetric liquid filling machine
6. Capping machine
7. Batch printing machine
8. Label gumming machine
9. Taping and sealing cartons
10. Digital balance.

36 In Process, Quality Control (QC) and Quality Assurance (QA) Tests of Pharmaceutical Products

In process, quality control tests are defined when the production of products is in process and has not reached the taping and sealing of cartons. Quality control is defined as satisfaction of label claim like potency, purity, pharmacological action, stability, uniformity of tests and hygienic environment. Quality is also a satisfied feedback from consumers. Quality assurance satisfies the standards of products. By control the quality, manufacturer can market products and produce reproduction of products easily. Four Ms leads to the quality of products.

1. Materials
2. Men
3. Machines
4. Methods

1. *Materials:* In this we have to purchase raw materials and receive raw materials clean and with gloves (Quarantine section). After physical examination and cleaning samples are tested and passes approval, unapproved raw materials are sent to manufacturer. After chemical test passes approval, raw materials are transferred to manufacturing with proper transaction of production records and labels. Similarly packing materials are tested and passes approval. Disapproved packing materials are sent to manufacturer. Raw materials and packing materials must not get destroyed by oxygen, air, moisture, heat and other external environment. Materials must be kept in shelves, labeled and packed. The bulk drugs bulk excipients and bulk packing materials must be protected from contamination.

2. *Men:* Men must be clean and clear about the quality of products. There must be no batch mixing. Weight and volume variation must be within the limits. The external

environment floor, windows, doors, roof, fans, etc. must be regularly clean. Labeling must be right. Zero defect in quality assurance. Thickness of tablets must be within limits.

3. *Machines:* Machines must be given highest output and low manpower use. Must be clean with isopropyl alcohol and regular use of mobilile and grease must be used. Machine must be clean with dry cloth. No batch mixing must take place and right labeling to be done. Right man should be assigned for right machine.

4. *Methods:* Methods used in processes, packing, etc. must contribute the yield and quality of products. Weight or volume variation, thickness variation, dissolution test, labeling and packing must be right as per the method prescribed in production records. Good manufacturing practices (GMP) must be used in proper production filling, tests uniformly conducted, right labeling and right packing is implemented and controls to obtain assured quality which gives satisfying results.

In case of uncoated and coated tablets, following observation must pass approval.

1. Appearance of tablets
2. Tablet thickness
3. Tablet diameter
4. Uniformity of weight variation
5. Tablet hardness
6. Tablet friability
7. Tablet surface
8. Tablet colour
9. Tablet polish
10. Strip pinhole test
11. Blister leak test
12. Disintegration test
13. Dissolution test

In case of hard or soft capsules, following observations must pass approval

1. Content of active ingredient
2. Uniformity of weight variation

3. Strip pin hole test
4. Blister leak test
5. Disintegration test
6. Dissolution test

In case of liquid orals, following tests must pass approval
1. Uniform volume variation
2. Dissolution test
3. Preservative
4. Solubility
5. Viscosity
6. Stability

In case of liquid parenterals, following tests must pass approval
1. Leak test
2. Sterility test
3. Uniform volume variation
4. Clarity test
5. Sealing test
6. Particulate matter absent

In case of creams, ointment, lotions, following tests must pass approval
1. Emulsification of oil and water phase
2. Microbiological test passes

Control Charts
These are used to explain the various processes which are to be implemented to obtain quality of products.

Quality Level
The upper and lower limits of average reading must be within the prescribed limit. If the limit is beyond the average reading, correction is to be done by control the average reading within the limits.

Laboratory
Laboratory performs certain chemical tests for quality of products.

Sampling

Sampling of raw materials, production or finished products is done to obtain overall quality control of products. For example 20 tablets or capsules are sampled to perform assay of products. 200 ml is sampled to perform assay of liquid orals. 200 ml is sampled to perform to assay creams, ointment, lotions, etc.

Common sampling is done once. Double or triple sampling is done when assay is not obtaining desired results.

Assay

Assay of all products is calculated, range from 90% to 110% and must be within the prescribed limits as per IP/BP/USP.

Stability

Stability of products is calculated up to its expiry date. Products must be stable at least up to expiry date. As per drugs and cosmetic Act 1940 all products and records must be stored up to 2 years from expiry date and products without expiry date must be stored up to 5 years from the date of manufacturing. All production records must be maintained and testing of products legally which may be recalled by the authority.

Chemical analysis, drug analysis, cosmetic analysis as per IP, BP, USP and FDA specifications. Microbiological test for cosmetics and non sterile products:

CFU = Colonies forming units

USP standard:

CFU = 30 to 300 CFU per plate

FDA standard:

CFU = 25 to 250 CFU per plate

Microbiological test for sterile products:

USP standard

CFU = 0 to 10 CFU per 100 ml

Sample in sample rooms are kept up to 1 year from date of expiry.

Records in record rooms are kept up to 1 year from date of expiry.

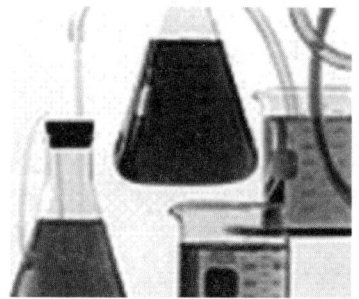

Solvent

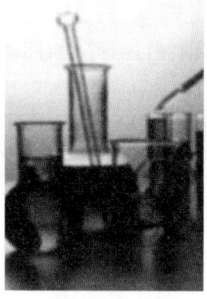

Chemical analysis

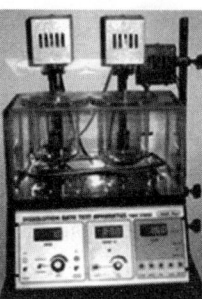

Dissolution test

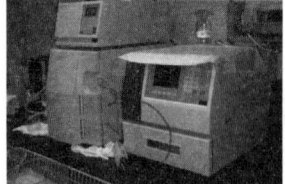

HPLC

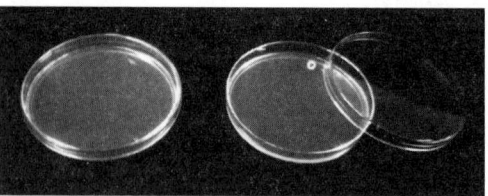

Agar plate

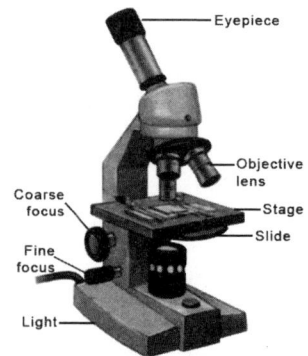

Microscope

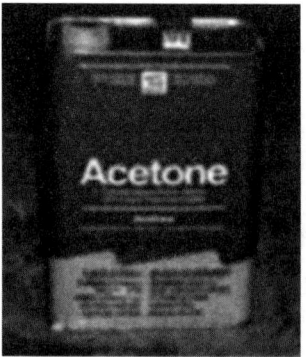

Solvent acetone

37 *Packing Technologies*

Packing of products is implemented because of following factors

1. Stability of products for example liquid fluids
2. Decontamination of products for example tablets, capsules
3. Dose of products for example ampoules
4. Easy selling for example tablets, capsules
5. Sterile for example ampoules, vials
6. Easy to carry for example tablets, capsules
7. Economical value for example capsule
8. Explain use of products for example cosmetics
9. Attract to shoppers attention for example colors

Conclusion of packing technologies is to protect the product retaining physical and chemical properties up to expiry date, safe in use, decontamination, economical saving and stability of products.

Liquid, liquid parenterals, strip, blister toothpaste, hair gel packing

1. Neutral glass
2. Transparent white glass bottles of borosilicate
3. Amber glass
4. Butyl rubber plugs
5. Aluminum seals
6. Plastic droppers
7. Plastic bottles
8. Plastic caps
9. Polyvinyl chloride and polyvinyl dichloride for plastic rolls for tablets and capsules
10. Plastic jars
11. Plastic tubes

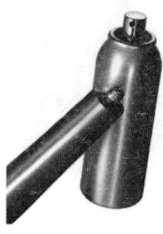
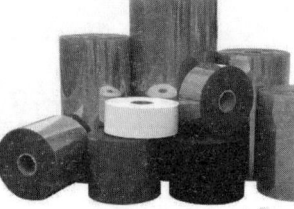
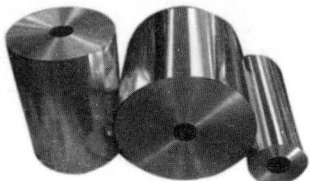

Aerosol can   Alu packing   Aluminium rolls

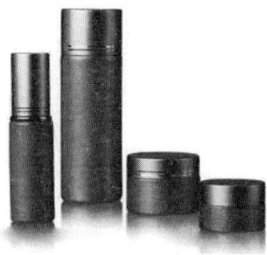
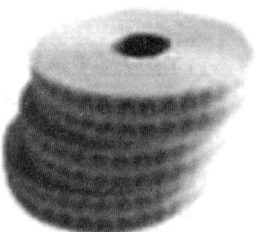

Cream jars   Paper pack

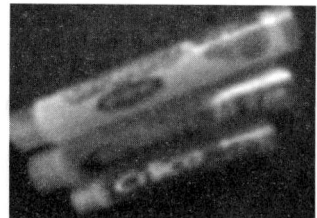
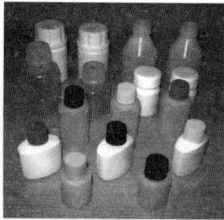
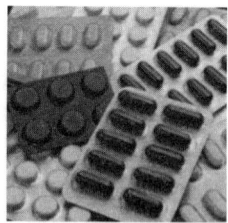

Plastic tubes   Plastic bottles   PVC/PDC pack

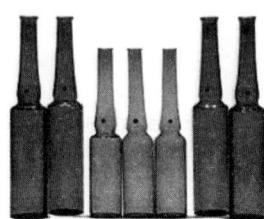
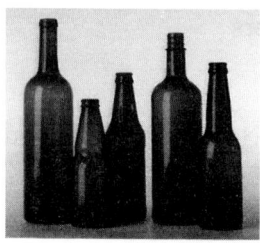
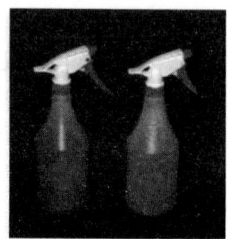

Ampoules   Soda lime glass bottles   Spray bottles

Metals for oils/strip, blister, alu pack

Generally aluminum containers are used. For strip, blister, alu pack for solids like tablets, capsules, thin printed aluminum rolls are used.

Paper Packing

Cellophane rolls are used for testing tablet, capsule machines running.

Aerosols Packing

Aerosols are used in perfumes, drugs packing. Aerosols container is made up of glass or plastic. Tetrafluorodichloroethane, trichloromonofluoromethane are used as propellants in aerosols in order to propel perfumes or drugs.

Strapping

Nylon and steel are used for straps.

Cartons

3 ply or 5 ply corrugated boxes are used in packing for proper transport of products.

38 Marketing

Analysis, planning, implementation and control of marketing formula. Marketing formula contain

1. *Most important ideas:* Consumers, products, prices, places, promotions, demands, needs, knowledge, belief, competitive industries, legal/regulatory acts, system constraints, ethical, technical.
2. *Important ideas:* Economic, social, cultural, information, strategic management.

Business is run by finance, production and marketing.

Company has finance $ 12 billion. Production capacity per month is 5000 metric tons. Marketing turnover is $ 12 crore annual. Company can make profits only when it produces high quality products, at low price and high quality products are right products as per the demand of consumers.

Consumption expenditure per day, per capita income in decreasing order:

1. Cement, electicity, water
2. Health food products
3. Fabric
4. Oil and gas
5. Computer/telephone/mobile
6. Auto
7. Ethanol
8. Cosmetics
9. Drugs
10. Cigarette

Cosmetic is growing @8% annual, drugs is growing @6% annual. Food products is growing @12% annual. Herbal products like liquid extracts, powders are growing @12% annual due to right products, homeopathic pharmacy is growing @10%, allopathic pharmacy growing @6% annual due to adverse reactions. Government should give high subsidy and loans without interest to promote ayurvedic pharmacy for the benefit of public and export business. HP and TN in India are the examples of ayurvedic pharmacy.

In this book I have written products which have demanded and are market leaders from thousands of years.

Actual example of price list of company A:

Brand	Product	Packing
Seczol	Paracetamol	500 mg Tablet
Distributor price	Rs. 5,417.28/-	Carton of 60 boxes
Wholesaler price	Rs.5, 472/-	Carton of 60 boxes of 10'S
Retailer price	Rs.9.60/-	10'S blister pack
MRP	Rs.12/-	10'S blister pack

In addition to price list deal 10% extra free with a box is delivered to retailers, with occussional gifts are delivered so that retailer can sell products.

39 *Name of Drugs Excipients*

Absorbents (Which absorb liquid)

- Bentonite
- Kaolin
- Magnesium carbonate
- Magnesium oxide
- Magnesium silicate
- Silica
- Starch
- Tricalcium phosphate

Antiadhesives (Antisticking agents)

- Magnesium stearate
- Talc

Antioxidants (Stops oxidation)

- Ascorbic acid
- Citric acid
- Glycerine
- Hydroquinone 4% w/w used for making white skin
- Maleic acid
- Vitamin E

Binders (Used in tablets wet granulation method)

- Acacia 1 to 2 % w/w in ayurvedic tablets
- Sodium carboxy methyl cellulose 2 to 3% w/w in homeopathatic tablets
- Polyvinylpyrrolidine K-30 2% w/w used in soluble and chewable tablets
- Maize starch used 3 to 5% w/w generally in allopathic tablets

Coating Materials (Used in Tablets)

- Cellulose acetate phthalate (soluble at pH>6, used in enteric coating of tablets)
- Hydroxypropyl methyl cellulose (soluble at pH<6, used in film coating)
- Polythylene glycols
- Sodium CMC high viscosity (used in film coating)
- Sugar (used in sugar coating)

Colours

- Natural colours
- Alizarin
- Caramel
- Beta carotene
- Carbon black
- Carmic acid
- Chlorophyll
- Curcumin
- Ferric oxides (red and yellow)
- Indigo
- Riboflavin
- Saffron
- Titanium dioxide
- Turmeric
- Tyrian purple
- Synthetic colours
- Alizarin cyanine
- Amaranth 1 N 16185
- Brillant blue FCS 42090
- Carmoisine 14720
- EosineG 45380
- Erthrosin 45430
- Fast red E 16045
- Fast green FCF 42053
- Green S 44090
- Green F 61570

- Indigo carmine 73015
- Naphthol blue black 20470
- Orange G 1630
- Ponceaux 4 R 16255
- Quinazarine 61565
- Quinoline yellow SS 47000
- Resorin brown 201700
- Sudan III 26100
- Sunset yellow FCF 15185
- Tartrazine 19140

Complexing Agents (Stops formation of bonds in formulation)

- Boric acid for glycerine
- Caffeine for organic acids, benzocaine, riboflavin
- Dextrins for vitamin A palmitate
- Sodium EDTA and Disodium EDTA for papaverine, morphine, vitamin C, antibiotics, epinephrine, prednisolone
- Sodium CMC for quinine, diphenhydramine, pyribenzamine
- PEG 400 for phenolos, barbiturates, organic acids, iodine protamine sulphate for heparin
- PVP K-30 for procaine HCl, salicylates, cortisones, xanthines
- Saccharin for phenolic compounds
- Surfactants like sodium lauryl sulphate for tablets

Diluents (Used in dilution)

- Calcium carbonate
- Dicalcium phosphate
- Sodium CMC food grade
- Lactose
- Magnesium carbonate
- Magnesium oxixe
- Mannitol PVP
- Maize starch
- Sucrose
- Sorbitol
- Tricalcium sulphate

Disintegrants (Breaking to form particals)

- Maize starch powder
- Reverse osmosis water

Dispersants (antiflocculants used to distribute small particles in liquid form)

- Sodium CMC 1% w/w
- Reverse osmosis water

Emulsifying agents (For mixing different phases)

- Castor oil
- PEG400
- PEG4000
- Propylene glycol
- Sodium lauryl sulphate
- Stearic acid
- Silica gel
- Triethanolmine

Flavouring Agents (Taste maker)

- Natural
- Please study appendixVI of essential oils
- Synthetic
- Almond
- Apricot
- Apple
- Banana
- Cheery
- Custurd
- Ginger
- Grape
- Jasmine
- Lemongrass
- Liquorice
- Mango
- Peach

- Pineapple
- Raspberry
- Sandalwood
- Strawberry
- Vanillin

Flocculating Agents (Formation of precipitates)
- Sodium chloride

Glidants (Free flow for dry granules)
- Maize starch
- Talc

Preservatives (To protect liquid from microorganisms)
- Benzalkonium chloride
- Methylparaben
- Propylparaben
- Sodium benzoate

Solubilising Agents (Dissolving solid and liquid phases)
- PEG400
- Sodium CMC
- Sadium lauryl sulphate

Solvents (Used in large quantity)
- Acetone 70%
- Ethanol
- PEG 400
- Propylene glycol
- Aqua

Suspending Agents
(solid particles are hanging in liquid phase)
- Sodium CMC
- Hydroxyl propyl cellulose PVP
- Pectin

Sweetening Agents (To make sweet taste)

- Dextrose
- Glycerine
- Honey
- Lactose
- Maltose
- Mannitol
- Saccharin
- Sorbitol
- Sucrose

Vehicles (Liquids)

- Ethyl alcohol
- Glycerine
- Mineral oil
- Polyethylene glycol
- Vegetable oils like mustard oil, corn oil, castor oil, olive oil, coconut oil

40 *Name of Cosmetics Ingredients*

Absorbents (Absorbs moisture)

- Calcium carbonate
- Maize starch
- Magnesium carbonate
- Tricalcium phosphate

Antiadhesives (Not sticking)

- Magnesium stearate
- Talc

Antioxidants (Stops oxidation)

- Vitamin A
- Vitamin C
- Vitamin E
- Butylated hydroxyanisole (BHA)
- Butylated hydroxytoluene
- Citric acid
- Hydroquinone
- Lecithin
- Maleic acid
- Sodium metabisulphite

Antiseptics (Inhibits germs)

- Benzalkonium chloride
- Boric acid
- Camphor
- Chlorhexidine diacetate
- Cinnamon oil
- Clove oil
- Menthol

- Methyl salicylate
- Phenol
- Salicylic acid
- Tannic acid

Antidandruff Agents
(removes white dead flakes on skin and hair)

- Camphor
- Neem oil
- Selenium sulphide
- Tea tree oil
- Zinc pyridinium
- Zinc undecylinate

Binders (Joining)

- Sodium CMC HV
- Hydroxypropyl cellulose
- Lanolin
- Mineral oil
- PVPK-30
- Maize starch

Colours

- Colours are explained in drugs excipients

Covering Agents (Coating)

- Kaolin
- Magnesium stearate
- Maize starch
- Talc
- Titanium dioxide
- Zinc oxide
- Zinc stearate

Detergents (Washing clothes/body)

- Coconut diethanolamide
- Sodium lauryl sulphate

Emollients (Softening)

- Cetyl alcohol
- Cocoa butter
- Groundnut oil
- Isopropyl myristate
- Lanolin
- Stearic acid

Film Formers (Thickner)

- Acacia
- Carbopol940
- Sodium CMCHV
- Sodium lauryl ether sulphate
- Lanolin
- Lanolin alcohol
- Lanolin oil
- Liquid paraffin
- Methacrylate
- Paraffin wax
- PVPK30
- Stearic acid

Hair Colourants (Colouring hair)

- Camomile
- Cobalt sulphate
- Cobalt sulphate
- Heena

Hair Removers (Removing hair from skin)

- Barium sulphide

Hair Conditioning Agents (Softening)

- Herbal extracts
- Lanolin
- Protein hydrolysate

Humectants (Moisturing)

- Fructose
- Glucose
- Glycerine
- Polyethylene glycol
- Polyoxyethylene sorbitol
- Propylene glycol
- Sodium lactate
- Triethylene glycol
- Triethanolamine
- Urea

Oils (Fat)

- Arachis oil
- Acetoglycerides
- Castor oil
- Essential oils
- Mustard oil
- Olive oil
- Paraffin oil
- Coconut oil
- Hydrogenated vegetable oils
- Isopropyl myristate
- Isopropyl palmitate
- Lonolin oil
- Peanut oil

Opacifiers (Brightness)

- Lithopone
- Titanium dioxide
- Zinc stearate

Pearlscent Agents (Brightness, shine)

- Almond oil
- Castor oil
- Liquid paraffin

- 4-methyl-7-diethylamino coumarin
- Mica
- Maize starch

Perfumes (Essence)

- Benzyl acetate
- Essential oils
- Phenyl ethyl alcohol

Plasticisers (Plastic)

- N-butyl stearate
- Castor oil
- Dibutyl phthalate
- Resorcinol diacetate
- Triethyl citrate
- Urea

Preservatives (Inhibits germs)

- Already explained in drug excipients.

Skin Nourishing Agents (Strength to skin)

- Fruit extracts
- Vitamin A
- Vitamin C
- Vitamin E

Solvents/Co solvents/Vehicles (Additives)

- Already explained in drug excipients

Sunscreen Agents

- Amyl salicylate
- Kaolin
- Magnesium oxide
- Calcium carbonate
- Para amino benzoic acid
- Phenyl salicylate
- Talc

Suntan Agents/Staining Agents (colour to skin)

- 8-Ethoxy psoralen
- Marigold
- Olive oil
- Walnut juice

Suspending Agents (Particle hanging in Liquid)

- Explained in drug excipients

Waxes (For creams, lotion, emulsion)

- White beeswax
- Cetyl alcohol
- Cetosteryl alcohol
- Cocoa butter
- Linolin
- Petroleum jelly
- Paraffin wax
- Petrolatum
- Stearic acid

100% Soluble Tablets of Lactose

The 50% v/v tincture when used with soluble tablets acts fast and patients feel healthier more quickly than with conventional tablets. Soluble tablets 100% dissolve in mouth while using. The quality of soluble tablets is best, working is best and price is economical. The number of soluble tablets are more than conventional tablets and are cylindrical shaped. These are prepared under hygienic environment, with gloves and not touched by hands. These are low in sugar and can be administered to diabetics. Such products are dispensed by homeopathic doctors.

Each uncoated tablet contains:
Ingredient:
Lactose = 42.18 mg, 66.43%

Excipients:
Starch=20.95 mg, 32.99%
Magnesium stearate = 0.19 mg, 0.3%

Lactose solube tablets

Average weight of 20 uncoated tablets = 63.49 mg
1 kg contains = 15,750 number of soluble tablets.

Pack: As per consumers needs

Antidote: Reverse osmosis water

Our main distributors of this product in UK is M/S House Of Mistry Limited, 15–17, South End Road, Hampstead London NW32PT, UK
E-mail: contact @ mistry.co.uk
Phone: 0044-1582-2077940848,
M/S GK Enterprises 33, Albion Road Luton, LU2ODS, UK
E-mail: ganju@hotmail.co.uk
Phone: 0044-1582-454528

100% pure herbal liquid extract, Environmentally friendly, No animal experiments!

Past History
It was used in ancient India for the internal and external body.

Description
It is a tree. Tree has roots, leaves, flowers, fruits and seeds. The fruit is circular in shape and brown in colour.

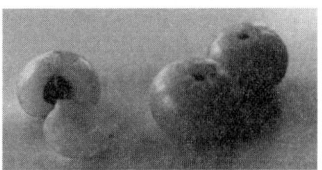
Fresh amla

Study of Emblica Extract
No adverse effect on the body. It can be used on any hair and/or skin type. Antidote is water.

Product Action
Well established for all kinds of hair wash, body wash and drinking emblica extract filtered for various remedies for example reduces body temperature, detoxifies the body, natural antioxidant.

The part used for emblica extract filter is the emblica fruit without its seed.

Chemical Analysis
The herbal extract contains Tannins. IT is a rejuvenating and natural antidandruff agent. It prevents arsenic damage to skin. The herbal extract is a rich source of vitamin C, bioflavonoid, and a natural anti-allergy mediator. This herbal extract also leaves the hair soft silky and manageable.

HDPL can also be used for calculations by percentage.

Product Range
• Shampoo

- Shampoo with conditioner
- Drinking product

It is used as one of the contents for preparation of herbal soaps in European countries.

Shampoo mixture of Sapindus Mukorossi, Acacia Concinna and Emblica are **available in the market.**

Direction of Use

The herbal extract is used for external and internal use. For the best results always dam the hair or body with water.

Packing Available

- **35 liters HDPE Jerry Canes**

Price: Rs. 84/- per litre.

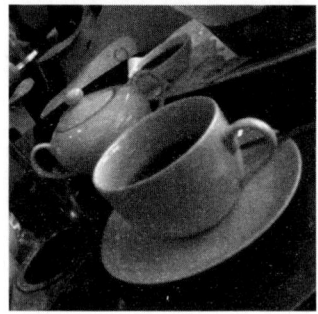

Liquid amla

100% pure herbal liquid extract, Environmentally friendly, No animal experiments!

Past History
It was used in ancient India for external body for washing.

Location
It grows in India.

Description
It is a tree. Tree has roots, leaves, flowers, fruits and seeds inside the fruits. The fruit is in rectangular shape. This fruit is brown in colour.

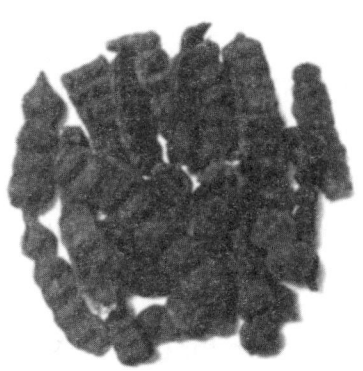

Shekakai

Part of Acacia Concinna Liquid used
Acacia concinna fruit without seed.

Study of Acacia Concinna Extract
No adverse effect in external body and hair is reported when the herbal extract is used. **Antidote** is water.

Product Action
Well established for hair wash, fabric wash, body wash, and skin.

Product Range
- Cleaning lotion
- Shampoo
- Shampoo with conditioner
- Detergent for any fabric
- Body wash
- Utensil cleaner

- Tile cleaner
- Shaving cream

It is used as one of the content for preparation of herbal soap in European countries. Shampoo with a mixture of sapindus mukorossi, acacia concinna and emblica is often used.

Chemical Analysis

The herbal extract containing saponins is responsible for its lather formation. It is used by shaking the liquid extract with water. Triterpenoidal prospogenols gives a natural bounce to the hair as well as softness to the hair. It makes any type of hair shinny, smooth, and dandruff free. It not only gives the skin soft effect but resorts the body's natural oils, thus free from skin diseases. It leaves the external body and any type of hair free from excess oiliness, dirt and lice. It is best for coloured and artificial hair. HPLC can be used for calculation by percentage.

Direction for use

The herbal extract is safe in used for external use. For best result of herbal extract always wet the body and hair.

Packing available

35 liters, HMHDPE Jerry Canes.

Price

Rs. 84 /- per litre.

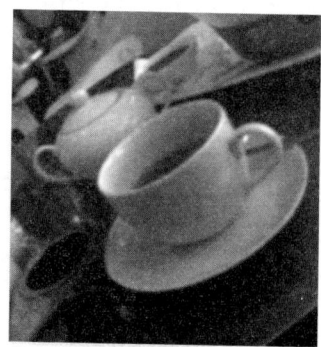

Liquid shekakai

IV 100% Dissolution Tablets of Lactose and Sucrose

The 50% v/v tincture when used with tablets acts fastest and consumers feel healthiest more quickly than with conventional tablets. Soluble tablets 100% gets dissolution in mouth while sucking, moving the tongue and chewing tablets within 1 minute. The quality of soluble tablets is best, working is best and price is very economical. The number of soluble tablets are more than conventional tablets, biconvex surface and round shaped. These are prepared under hygienic environment, with gloves and not touched by hands. These are low in sugar and can be administered to diabetes. Such products are dispensed by homeopathic doctors.

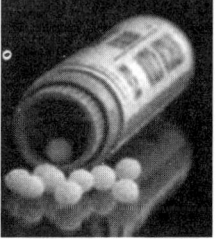

Crushed tablets are used as sweetening agent in tea, coffee, liquid fluids.

In process, quality control, quality assurance tests passes approval.

Dissolution tablets

Each White Film Coated Tablet Contains
Ingredient:
Lactose = 93.46 mg, 95.54%
Sucrose = 0.93 mg, 0.95%

Excipients:
Sodium carboxymethyl cellulose = 0.75 mg, 0.76%
Talcum = 0.89 mg, 0.92%
Magnesium stearate = 1.79 mg, 1.83%
Thickness of round tablet: 3 mm
Diameter of round tablet: –6.5 mm
Weight variation: –97.83 mg + –5%
Hardness: –4 kg/cm^2

Friability: Not more than 0.8% w/w

Average weight of 20 coated tablets = 97.83 mg

1 kg contains = 10,222 number of soluble tablets

Surface area of round tablet = 61.28 square mm

Volume of round tablet = 99.59 cubic mm

Disintegration time in machine= 30 minutes

Dissolution time in machine= 45 minutes

Tablet formulation is safe for pediatrics', adults, geriatrics, breastfeeding and pregnancy because crushed tablets make transparent solution in water due to ingredients and excipients.

Pack
As per consumers needs in drums.

Price
Rs. 500/- per kg

Antidote
Reverse osmosis water.

Our main distributors of this product in UK is M/S House of Mistry Limited, 15–17, South End Road, Hampstead London NW32PT, UK

E-mail: contact@mistry.co.uk

Phone: 0044-1582-2077940848.

Sapindus Mukorossi Product Literature

100% pure herbal liquid extract, Environmentally friendly, No animal experiments!

Past History
It was used in ancient India as liquid soap for hair wash and any type of fabric wash.

Location
It grows in India.

Description
It is a tree. The tree has leaves, flowers, fruits, root and seeds. The fruit is almost circular in shape and brown in colour.

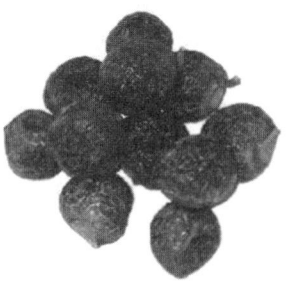

Reetha with seed inside

Part of Sapindus Mukorossi used for Extract Filtered
Sapindus Mukorossi fruit without seeds. The liquid extract filtered is brown in colour.

Study
This product can be used on the external body. The **antidote** is water.

Product Action
Well established for all kinds of hair wash, body wash, and all type of washing fabrics and effective for light brown spot on skin usually by exposure in the sun.

Product Range
- Cleansing lotion
- Shampoo
- Shampoo with conditioner
- Detergent for any fabric

- Body wash
- Utensil cleaner
- Floor cleaner
- Shaving cream

It is used as one of the content for preparation of herbal soap in European countries. Shampoo with a mixture of sapindus mukorossi, acacia concina and emblica is available in the market.

Chemical Analysis

The herbal extract filtered contains saponins, which is responsible for its lather formation. It is used either by shaking with water or by massaging the extract on the hands. Poly saccharides give a soft feel to the skin and hair. It helps the external body and any type of hair to stay free from excessive oiliness, dirt and lice. HPLC can be used for calculation in percentage.

Direction for Use

The herbal liquid extract filtered is safe for external use. For the best result the body and hair must always be wet.

Packing Available

35 liters HMH.DPE Jerry Canes.

Price

Rs. 84/- per litre. Transport extra.

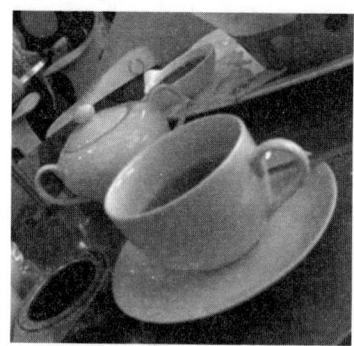

Liquid extract reetha

Sunny Enterprises
Essential Oils

From Ancient to Modern Therapy

The use of essential oils by Romans during ancient times is evident when they have used tons of oils in meals, bath and for pleasant effect. During modern therapy its use is added to perfume and aromatherapy.

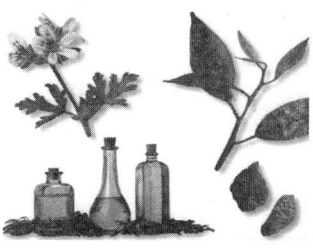

Essential oil

Aromatherapy is useful in stress management, headaches, colds, fever, muscular pain and pregnancy. Aromatherapy is a system in which body's natural strength is balanced, healed and maintained by the use of essential oils.

How can you use Essential Oils?

In the bath: Add 5 to 6 drops of essential oil in a full bucket of water and mix with clean hands. You can now take a bath which will give you pleasant feeling.

Room freshener: Add few drops of essential oil in the cotton. Place the cotton in the room. Essential oils perfume will create a fresh aromatic smell in the room.

In massage: Add 5 to 10 ml of essential oil to 10 ml of base oil. Shake the mixture thoroughly to blend before use. Test on small area of skin for sensitivity before using.

In cooking: Essential oils are very strong. Add only one drop to salad oil or vinegar. Use very sparingly.

Inhalation: Add few drops to your favourite cream, cleanser or lotion, shampoo. Blend thoroughly before use. Never apply undiluted essential oil directly to skin (with the exception of lavender oil).

As a perfume: Mix into base oil to create your own personal perfume.

In oil burner: To create a wonderful aromatic atmosphere in your home, try using an oil burner. With water in the bowl add 3 to 4 drops of your favourite essential oil light the candle and enjoy.

Essential oils are diluted between half to three percent depending on persons skin, the area to be treated, the age of those being massaged, the strength of the essential oil used and the condition for which it is being used. Don't exceed a two percent concentration on the facial massage. Start with one percent and step up to next concentration if the skin shows no redness or irritation.

Normally you don't need to go beyond two and a half percent but where there is great deal of muscular tension then three percent concentration of essential oil in the carrier oil (3 drops in 5 ml) could be used for a short period.

A message with aromatherapy oils should not be continued beyond a twelve week period, when there should be a break. It may be carried out on the alternate days where the condition is troublesome and when the improvement is felt, then reduced to twice a week then gradually to once a week.

If larger quantities of oil are required, then fill a 50 ml dark glass bottle (not plastic) with a base oil, then add the required essential oil.

Half percent concentration = 5 ml of essential oil + 50 ml base oil.
One percent concentration = 10 drops of essential oil + 50 ml base oil.
Two percent concentration = 20 drops of essential oil + 50 ml base oil

These oils can be stored in a cool dark place but should be used within a couple of months or they will loose their therapeutic value.

Essential Oils should be stored in a cool dark place and undiluted will keep the essence of their therapeutic value up to three years.

Precautions with Essential Oils

- During pregnancy check with professional/doctor before using essential oils.
- Never take essential oils internally.
- Avoid contact with eyes and other sensitive areas.

- Should you suffer an adverse reaction to any essential oil stop using it immediately.
- If you suffer from a medical condition (high blood pressure, epilepsy, etc.) check with the physician before using essential oils.
- Never use essential oils undiluted on the skin.
- Never use essential oil on babies or small children except under professional guidance.
- Antidotes are purified water and any range of soap.

Essential oils are extracted from plants and are highly concentrated and completely pure. Essential oils have many uses and are pleasurable to use. They should be used with care; always dilute them in base oil.

Aniseed
It helps to ease the tension, nervous headaches. Add to bath to ease headaches and tension. Also used in cases of bronchitis and colic. Used to flavor cooking. Aids digestion. Sweet and fruity odour. Uplifting.

Bergamot
Blends well with camomile, clary-sage, mandarin orange or neroli. Avoid going into sunshine for two hours after a massage with this oil.

Carrayway
Antimicrobial helps in cases of colic and bronchitis.

Cedarwood
Mild, balsamic-woody odour. Treats oily skin, oily hair and also mucossy coughs and colds.

Cinnamon
Powerful antiseptic used in inhalation in cases of colds and flu. Useful to relief flatulence and colic. Avoid in pregnancy.

Clove
Strong antiseptic. Diluted, makes a useful mouthwash or gargle with eucalyptus. Has an analgesic effect on gums.

Eucalptus

Use as an inhalation or blend with oils of lavender, pine and thyme when breathing is obstructed by cold. Massage into chest. Freshens sick rooms.

Fennel

Used in gargles. Calming. Aids digestion.

Jasmine

Expensive. Only used in tiny amounts. Anti depressant. Relieves menstrual pain. Relaxing and emotionally stimulating.

Juniper

Cleansing. Excellent in massage oil to relieve rheumatism.

Lavender

The most useful oil. Only oil that can be used undiluted. Use in undiluted form straight onto burns (as long as skin is not broken). Soothes bruises. Painkiller. Useful as an antiseptic, as an insect repellant. Aids relaxation and sleep. Calming.

Lemon

Invigorating. Refreshing. Stimulating. Useful on insect bites and stings. Do not add to baths, may cause burning sensation on skin. Astringent and cleaning.

Lemongrass

Antibacterial. Makes a good foot bath. Sweet and lemony. Good room freshner.

Neroli

Orange blossom. Calming and uplifting. Blends well with clary-sage, bergamot, lavender and camomile.

Patchouli

Musky, intriguing fragrance. Uplifting and stimulating. Added to water it makes a good rinse for excessively oily hair.

Pine

Invigorating. Makes a good steam inhalation. Combate lethargy (in a bath). Aids breathing. Helpful in bronchitis and respiratory problems. Use cautiously in babies, infants and children.

Rosemary

Stimulating. Good, useful, all around. Aids concentration. Dispels lethargy, especially Monday morning feeling. Improves circulation. Useful in colds. Improves bowel movement (constipation). Helps dandruff. Improves hair growth in daldness. Use in small quantities in babies and children. Use in migraine or a hangover. Helps to relieve aching muscles. Do not use in pregnancy.

Rose Otto

Cleansing. Purifies physically and emotionally. Helpful in addiction and allergies.

Rosa centifolia/damascene

Headache and migraine (due to allergy) hangover PMT especially good for mature skin. Mentally it supports and eases worry about the past, regret, sadness, fear, grief and attachment. Extremely useful oil. Rather expensive. Do not use on babies and infants.

Sandalwood

Expression/self expression. Useful for the skin especially throat area. Use for catarrh, bronchitis, sore throat, hoarseness. Also sinusitis, bronchitis, loss of voice, coughing. Helpful in cystitis. Useful in dry eczema. Treats skin eruptions such as carbuncles. Eases tinnutis. Psychologically it support negative feelings such as insecurity and worry about the future. Fear of coming events. Recurrent dreams. Listless and dread of making an effort. In meditation it aids sensivity and intuition.

Tea Tree

Antiseptic. Powerful immune system stimulant. Antifungual, antibacterial. Suitable to treat acne, candida, mouth ulcers, thrush and veruccae. Strong antibiotic. Use with extreme caution on babies and infants.

Ylang-Ylang

Especially useful in instilling confidence. Psychological conditions such as irritability, panic attacks, anger, fear of people or of failure. Guilt. Jealousy. Aids self esteem and self confidence. Helps shyness.

Exposure to Sun

Do not go out into the sun for three hours after using bergamot, grapefruit, lemon, lime and orange.

Babies, children and sensitive skin: Do not use on children under 2 years old; citronella, lemongrass and melissa.

Natural Essential Oils

Common	Latin	Country of origin	10 ml/ pound
Aniseed	Illicium verum	China	1.50
Basil	Ocimum basilicum	France	2.50
Bay	Pimenta racemosa	West Indies	2.50
Bergamot	Citrus bergamia	Ivory Coast/ Italy	2.50
Black Pepper	Piper nigrum	India	3.50
Cajaput	Melaleuca cajaput	Indonesia	1.50
Camphor	Cinnamomum Camphora	India	1.50
Cardamon	Elettaria cardamomum	India	3.50
Cedarwood	Cedrus deodorata	India	1.50
Chamomile	Ormensis multicaulis	Morocco	6.50
Cinnamon	Cinnamomum zeylancium	India	1.50
Citronella	Cymbopogon nardus	India	1.50
Clary Sage	Salvia sclarea	France	3.50
Clove Leaf	Eugenia caryophyllata	India	3.50
Cypress	Cupressus sempervirens	Austria	3.50

Eucalyptus	Eucalyptus globus	India	1.50
Fennel sweet	Foeniculum vulgare	Italy/ hungary	1.50
Geranium	Pelargonium graveolens	China	3.50
Ginger	Zingiber officinalis	India	3.50
Grapefruit	Citrus paradisi	Israel	1.50
Ho Leaf	Cinnamomum camphora	China/ South America	2.50
Hyssop	Hyssopus officinalis	France	3.50
Juniper Berry	Juniperus Communis	Croatia	3.50
Lavender	Lavendula angustifolium	France/China	2.00
Lemon	Citrus limonum	India	1.50
Lemongrass	Cymbopogon citratus	India	1.50
Lime	Citrus aurantifolia	Mexico	2.50
Mandarin	Citrus nobilis	Italy	2.50
Marjoram	Thymus masticina	Spain	3.50
Melissa	Melissa officinalis	UK blend	4.50
Myrrh	Comiphora myrrha	French distillation	5.50
Nutmeg	Myristica fragrans	India	2.50
Orange sweet	Citrus Cinesis	India	1.50
Palmarosa	Cymbopogon martini	Comores/ brasil	2.50
Patchouli	Pogostemon patchouli	Indonesia	2.50
Peppermint	Mentha piperata	India	1.50

Pine	Pinus sylvestris	Various	2.50
Rose geranium	Blend		3.50
Rosemary	Rosmarinus officinalis	Spain/tunisia	1.50
Sage	Salvia officinelis	Spain	3.50
Sandelwood	Santalum album	India	7.50
Spearmint	Mentha spicata	USA	1.50
Tangerine	Citrus reticulata	Spain/China	2.50
Thyme	Thymus vulgaris	India	1.50
Tea-tree	Melaleuca alternifolia	Australia	3.50
Wintergreen	Gaultheria procumbens	USA	1.50
Ylang-Ylang	Cananga odorata	Comores	3.50

Pure essential oils 10 ml, budget price pound 1.50 each

Base Oil Fixed Oil Budget Price

	10 ml (in pounds)	50 ml (in pounds)
Almond oil	1.50	2.50
Arnica	1.50	2.50
Avocado	1.50	2.50
Chickweed	1.50	2.50
Evening primrose	2.50	5.50
Grapeseed	1.50	2.50
Jojoba	2.50	5.50
Marigold	1.50	2.50
Olive	1.50	2.50
Vitamin E	2.50	5.50
Wheatgerm	1.50	2.50

Plain massage oils 50 ml budget price pound 2.50 each

Plain massage oil, massage oil with rose, massage oil with rosemary, massage oil with lavender, massage oil with tea-tree, massage oil with lemon, massage oil with juniper.

Note:

1. As desired we are the importers and exporters at present to UK and India products like essential oils, walnuts, Kashmir dry fruits and Kashmir handicrafts.
2. Please let us know if you can send some items for India market.
3. Essential oils can be send in bulk quantity in aluminium, etc. as per you need.

For sales and further information please contact us now:
Sunny Enterprises, 171, Puran Nagar, PO Lane, New Plots, Jammu–180005, Jandk State, India.
E-mail: Ranjan.magazine@Gmai.com,
Ph: 00-91-191-2579210; *Mobile:* 9797655365

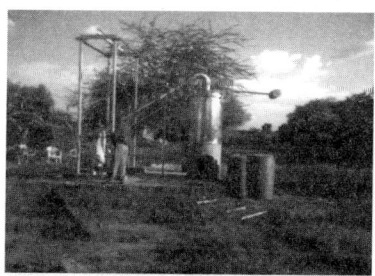
Essential oil distillation

VII Price Calculation of Film Coated Tablets

MRP calculation per batch = Cost price of packing + Cost price of manpower + Cost price of raw materials + Overhead 30% + Profit 20%

Cost price of bulk packing HMHDPE20 KG

1. HMHDPE drums 20 kg capacity = Cost of drum Rs. 195/- + Rate of duty 8% = Rs. 195/- = Rs. 15.60/- = Rs. 211/- (round number)
   Total Rs. = 211/-
   CED @8% Rs. = Rs.16.88/-
   Cess @2% Rs. = 0.34/-
   H Edu Cess @1% Re. 0.17/-
   Sub total Rs.= 230/-
   CST/VAT @2% Rs. 4.60/-
   Freight/transport Rs. 45/-
   Total Rs. 280/- is equivalent to 20 kg packing

2. 50 kg polythene bag @Rs. 100/- per kg (10 pieces) = Rs. 10/- per piece

3. Cost of 1 kg bag @Rs. 200/- per kg (80 pieces) = Rs. 2.50/ per piece = Rs. 2.50/- * 20 Rs. 50/- per drum.

4. Cost of rubber band = Re. 1/- per piece = Rs.1*21 = Rs.21/- per drum

5. Cost of 500 grams cotton @ Rs. 125/- per kg = Rs. 63/- per drum

6. Aluminum wire sealing = Rs. 5/- per drum
   Sub cost price for 20 kg packing = Rs. 429/-
   Sub total cost price for 1 kg packing = Rs. 22/-

Cost Price of Manpower

Manager Rs. 15, 000/- + worker Rs. 4, 000/- = Rs.19, 000/- for 24.50 working days, 8 hourly

Total working days   = 15 (manual grinding)

Total working hours   = 15*8 = 120 hours

Rs. 97/- for 1 hour work

Cost of 120 hours work   = Rs. 97/- *120 = Rs. 11,640/-

Rs. 11,640/- for 17 kg batch

Rs. 685/- for 1 kg batch (manual grinding)

Cost price of manpower = Rs. 685/- for 1 kg batch

Cost Price of Bulk Raw Materials (500 kg)

1. Cost of lactose per kg for 500 kg batch = Cost of lactose Rs. 66/- + CED Rs. 4.50/- per kg = Rs.70.50/- per kg + CST 2% = Rs. 70.50/- + Rs. 1.41/- = Rs. 72/- per kg
2. Cost of sodium CMC high viscosity 25 kg bag = Cost of CMC Rs. 150/- + CST/2% = Rs. 150/- + Rs. 3/- = Rs. 153/- per kg
3. Cost of talcum powder 25 kg bag = Rs. 12/- + CST 2% = Rs. 12 + Rs. 0.24/- = Rs. 13/- per kg
4. Cost of magnesium stearate per kg for 25 kg bag = Rs. 72/- CED Rs. 5.48/- per kg = Rs. 78/- + CST 2%= Rs. 78/- + Rs. 1.56/- = Rs. 80/- per kg
5. Cost of sucrose = Rs. 55/- per kg
6. Forwarding charges = Rs. 100/- *4 = Rs. 400/-
7. *Freight and transport:* Rs. 7.50/- *550 kg = Rs.4,125/-, local for 550 kg = Rs.500/-

Freight and Transport for 500 kg Raw Materials = Rs. 5,000/-
Formula

1. Lactose = 18,000 gm
2. Sucrose = 180 gm
3. Sodium CMC HV = 144 gm
4. Talcum = 172.52 gm
5. Magnesium stearate = 345.04 gm

Total weight = 18,841.56 gm which is equivalent to 17 kg of finished product

1. Cost of 18,000 gm of lactose = Rs. 72/- * 18 = Rs.1,296/-
2. Cost of 180 gm of sucrose = Rs. 40*180/1000 = Rs. 7.20/-
3. Cost of 144 gm of sodium CMC HV = Rs. 153*144/1000 = Rs. 23/-
4. Cost of 173 gm of talcum = Rs. 13/- *173/1000 = Rs. 3/-
5. Cost 346 gm of magnesium stearate = Rs. 80/- *346/1000 = Rs. 32/-
6. Forwarding charges for 19 kg = Rs. 100/-
7. Freight and transport for 19 kg = Rs. 190/-

Cost price for 17 kg = Rs. 1662/-

Cost price for 1 kg = Rs. 98/-

Total cost price = Cost price of packing Rs. 22/- + Cost price of manpower Rs. 685/- + Cost price of raw materials Rs. 98/- = Rs.805/-

Overhead per 1 kg @ 30% = Rs. 242/-

Profit per 1 kg @ 20% = Rs. 210/-

MRP per 1 kg = Rs. 805/- + Rs. 242/- +Rs. 210/- = Rs. 1, 257/-

No. of tablets in 1 kg = 10,221

MRP per 1 tablet = Rs. 1, 257/10221 = 12.30 paise only

Note:
1. Calculation is based on 500 kg order
2. Local transport, insurance goods and sea cargo charges extra as per actual.

MRP Calculation of Liquid Extract Reetha

Cost of raw materials + cost of manpower + cost of packing + overhead 30% + profit 25.37%

1. Cost of reetha 5 kg @ Rs. 70/- per kg = Rs. 350/-
2. Cost of reverse osmosis water 60 litres @ Re. 1/- per litre = Rs. 60/-
3. Cost of sodium benzoate for 50 litres extract is 25 gm (0.05% w/v) @ Rs. 100/- per kg = Rs. 5/-
4. Cost of 3 heaters for 60 litres @ Rs. 40/- per heater = Rs. 120/-
5. Cost of wastage disposal of 5 kg @ Rs. 20/- per kg = Rs. 100/-
6. Worker/management cost for 35 litres net for 1 day (8 hours) = Rs. 700/-
7. Cost of HMHDPE Jerry Canes 35 litres = Rs. 430/-
8. Cost of gloves/soap/powder/gumming/labels = Rs. 2/- + Rs. 2/- + Rs. 2/- + Rs. 2/- + Rs. 5/- = Rs. 15/-
9. Cost price for 35 litres = Rs. 1,780/-
10. Cost price of 1 litre = Rs. 51/-
11. Overhead 30% = Rs. 16/- (round number)
12. Total cost price per 1 litre = Rs. 67/-
13. Profit 25.37% = Rs. 16.99/- per litre
14. MRP per 1 litre = Rs. 84/-

Note: Local, road, insurance goods, sea cargo extra. Minimum order for quantity = 2,000 litres.

Appendix IX Sunny Enterprises Labels

Name of Product:

Batch no.:

Quantity:

Shipper: M/s Sunny Enterprises
171 Puran Nagar, PO Lane, New Plots, Jammu-180005, India.

I.E. code no.: 1894000781

Date of issue: 13-2-1995, **Pan:** AEXPM9502N

To

Liquid Extracts and Extracts

1. Amla (Emblica)
Chemical analysis: Nutritional, vitamin C
Uses: Used in shampoo, cream, juice, paste, dry powder, capsule of fruit part.

2. Neem Leaves (Azadirachta Indica)
Chemical analysis: Antiseptic, antimicrobial
Uses: Used in shampoo, cream, juice, paste, dry powder, capsule of leave, stem part.

3. Jatamansi (Nardostachys jatamansi)
Chemical analysis: Antianxiety producing sleep.
Uses: Used in shampoo, cream, juice, paste, dry powder, capsule of root and rhizomes part.

4. Brahmi (Bacopa monnieri)
Chemical analysis: Antioxidant, increases memory
Uses: Used in shampoo, creams, juice, paste, dry powder, capsule of leaves and stems part.

5. Methi (Trigonella foenum-graecum)
Chemical analysis: Contains proteins and amino acids.
Uses: Used in shampoo, cream, juice, dry powder, capsule of leaves, stem, seeds part.

6. Tulsi (Ocimum sanctum)
Chemical analysis: Nutritional
Uses: Used in shampoo, cream, juice, paste, dry powder, capsule of stem and leaves part.

7. Kapur Kachari (Hedychium spicatum)
Chemical analysis: Glucosides for strength
Uses: Used in shampoo, cream, juice, paste, dry powder, capsule of root and rhizomes part.

8. **Chandan (Santalum album)**
   Chemical analysis: Perfume
   Uses: Used in shampoo and creams of wood part.

9. **Ghritkumari (Aloe barbadensis)**
   Chemical analysis: Amino acids, vitamins, minerals, saponins, enzyme and polysaccharides
   Uses: Used in shampoo, cream, juice, paste or dry powder of plant.

10. **Harida (Amragandhi)**
    Chemical analysis: Tannins for colour and taste.
    Uses: Used in shampoo, cream, juice, paste or dry powder of root, leaves, stem part.

11. **Hriber (Rouwolfia sepentina)**
    Chemical analysis: Alkaloids producing sleep
    Uses: Used in shampoo, cream, juice, paste or dry powder, capsule of root, leaves, stem part.

12. **Kadir (Pogostemon cablin)**
    Chemical analysis: Perfume
    Uses: Used in shampoo, cream of leaves part.

13. **Kumud (Nymphaea nouchali)**
    Chemical analysis: Antidiabetics, treat indigestion
    Uses: Used in shampoo, cream, juice, paste, dry powder, capsule of rhizomes, leaves, stem part.

14. **Bhavprakash (Crocus sativus)**
    Chemical analysis: Colorant
    Uses: Used in shampoo, cream of dry flowers

15. **Rastarangini (Shankhadrav)**
    Chemical analysis: Glycosides for strength
    Uses: Used in shampoo, cream, juice, paste, dry powder, capsule of leaves, e.g. Shilajit

16. **Liquorice (Glycyrrhiza)**
    Chemical analysis: Contains potassium, calcium salts, and saponins.
    Uses: Used in shampoo, creams, juice, paste, dry powder, capsule of roots.

17. **Shatvari (Asparagus racemosus)**
    Chemical analysis: Saponins, glycoside for strength.
    Uses: Used in shampoo, cream, juice, paste, dry powder, capsule of roots, leaves, stem.

18. **Ashwaganda (Withania somnifera)**
    Chemical analysis: Phenol for taste and smell, glycoside for strength.
    Uses: Used in shampoo, cream, juice, paste, dry powder, capsule of roots.

19. **Vidarikand (Pueraria tuberose)**
    Chemical analysis: Starch, alkaloid for sleep, potassium salts
    Uses: Used in shampoo, creams, juice, paste, dry powder, capsule of roots.

20. **Kaunch beej (Mucuna pruriens)**
    Chemical analysis: Proteins, fibres
    Uses: Used in shampoo, creams, juice, paste, dry powder, capsule of seeds and roots.

21. **Varahik (Dioscorea bulbifera)**
    Chemical analysis: Starch, glycosides for strength
    Uses: Used in shampoo, cream juice, paste, dry powder, capsule of rhizomes

22. **Suddha Shilajit (asphalt)**
    Chemical analysis: Salts of calcium, magnesium.
    Uses: Used in shampoo, cream, juice, paste, dry powder, capsule of bark, seeds, roots and leaves.

23. **Pippali (Piper longum)**
    Chemical analysis: Perfume
    Uses: Used in shampoo, cream, of fruit

24. **Ginseng (Pinax ginseng)**
    Chemical analysis: Saponins, nutritional
    Uses: Used in shampoo, cream, juice, paste, dry powder, capsule of roots and leaves.

25. **Ginkgo biloba (Ginkgo biloba)**
    Chemical analysis: Glycosides for strength, vitamin C.
    Uses: Used in shampoo, cream, juice, paste, dry powder, capsule of leaves.

26. **Jatifal (Myristica fragnans)**
    Chemical analysis: Proteins, carbohydrate fiber, fats, salts of calcium and phosphorus for strength
    Uses: Used in shampoo, cream, juice, paste, dry powder, capsule of stem, bark, leaves, flowers.

27. **Garlic (Allium sativum)**
    Chemical analysis: Amino acids, sulphur, allin
    Uses: Used in shampoo, cream, juice, paste, dry powder, capsule of bulb.

28. **Reetha (Sapindus murrossi)**
    Chemical analysis: Saponins for cleaning body.
    Uses: Used in shampoo of fruit.

29. **Shekakai (Acacia Concinna)**
    Chemical analysis: Saponins for cleaning body.
    Uses: Used in shampoo of fruit part.

30. **Arjuna bark (Terminalia arjuna)**
    Chemical analysis: Saponins, salts of calcium, magnesium, zinc, copper.
    Uses: Used in shampoo, cream, juice, paste, dry powder, capsule of stem, bark, leaves.

31. **Sarasaparilla (Hemidesmus indicus)**
    Chemical analysis: Saponins, antimicrobial
    Uses: Used in shampoo, cream, juice, paste, dry powder, capsule of leaves, roots.

32. Soap lily (Chlorogalum pomeridianum)
Chemical analysis: Saponins for cleaning body.
Uses: Used in shampoo.

33. Ashoka (Saraca indica)
Chemical analysis: Tannins for taste and colour, salts of calcium, antibacterial, antifungal, saponins
Uses: Used in shampoo, cream, juice, paste, dry powder, capsule of stem, bark, flowers, leaves.

34. Lodhra (Symplocos racemosa)
Chemical analysis: Glycosides for strength
Uses: Used in shampoo, cream, juice, paste, dry powder, capsule of leaves, bark.

35. Kantikari (Solanum ferox)
Chemical analysis: Alkaloids for sleep.
Uses: Used in shampoo, cream, juice, paste, dry powder, capsule of roots, leaves, stems, flowers, fruits and seeds.

36. Gokshura (Tribulus terrestris)
Chemical analysis: Saponins
Uses: Used in shampoo, cream, juice, paste, dry powder, capsule of leaves, stems, fruits and roots.

37. Marigold (Calendula officinalis)
Chemical analysis: Antibiotics, antiseptic, antiviral, analgesic, antifungal, antiinflammatory, antiage, antioxidant, lutein, zeaxanthin.
Uses: Used in shampoo, creams of flowers part.

38. Seena (Cassia angustifolia)
Chemical analysis: Used in shampoo, cream, juice, paste, dry powder, capsule of leaves, stems.

39. Turmeric (Curcuma Longa Linn)
Chemical analysis: Tannins for colour and taste.
Uses: Used in shampoo, cream, paste, dry powder of root.

40. **Kirayat (Andrographis paniculata)**

    Chemical analysis: Phenol, tannins for colour and taste, saponins.

    Uses: Used in shampoo, cream, juice, paste, dry powder, capsule of leaves and roots.

41. **Hari taki (Terminalia chebula)**

    Chemical analysis: Phenolic for colour and taste, flavonoid as antioxidant, anti-inflammatory, carotenoid as antioxidant.

    Uses: Used in shampoo, cream, juice, paste, dry powder, capsule of fruits, leaves, stems.

42. **Kava kava (Pipermethysticum)**

    Chemical analysis: Alkaloids for sleep.

    Uses: Used in shampoo, cream, juice, paste, dry powder, capsule of leaves, stem part.

43. **Baehra (Terminalia bellirica)**

    Chemical analysis: Saponins, glycosides

    Uses: Used in shampoo, cream, juice, paste, dry powder, capsule of leaves and stem.

Bibliography

1. A. Wade and PJ Weller. Handbook of Pharmaceutical Excipients, 2nd edition, American Pharmaceutical Association, Washington, 1994.
2. A.L. Gennaro. Remington's Pharmaceutical Sciences, 18th edition, Mark Publishing Company, Pennsylvania, 1990.
3. British Pharmaceutical Codex, 11th and 12th editions, The Pharmaceutical Press, London, 1994.
4. British Pharmacopoeia. Office of British Pharmacopoeia Committee, London, 1988.
5. Indian Pharmacopoeia, 2nd, 3rd, and 4th editions, the Controller of Publications, Delhi, 1966, 1985 and 1996.
6. Leon Lachman, HA, Lieberman. The Theory and Practice of Industrial Pharmacy, 3rd edition, Varghese Publishing House, Bombay, 1987.
7. SJ Carter, Copper and Gunns. Dispensing for Pharmaceutical Students, 12th edition, Pitman Medical Publishing Co. Ltd., Kent, 1975.
8. United States Pharmacopoeia, 23 and NF 18, Asian Edition, U.S. Pharmacopocial Convention, Inc. 1995.
9. Hoover. Dispensing of Medication, 8th edition, Mack Publishing Company, Pennsylvania, 1976.
10. Lieberman, HA and Lachman, L Tablets, volume 1 to 3, Marcel Dekker, New York.
11. Drugs and Cosmetics Act 1940 and Rules 1945, Govt of India Publication.
12. Extra Pharmacopoeia Martindale
13. National Formulary of India
14. Anne Young. Practical Cosmetic Science, Mills and Boon Ltd., London, UK.

15. rankandco@vsnl.net, www.dhimanindia.com for Pharmacy Machines

16. www.google.com

17. Drug Index. Passi Publication, 2010

18. Textbook of Pharmacognosy. CBS Publications and Distributors, New Delhi, Mohammed Ali.

Index

Reader's Notes

Reader's Notes

Reader's Notes